Chest X-rays
for Medical Students

Christopher Clarke
To my parents, Carole and David, and brothers
William and Nicholas

Anthony Dux
To my wife, Sally, and children Emma and Marcus
And to Dr Joe Gleeson who started me off in radiology

Chest X-rays
for Medical Students

Christopher Clarke
Specialty Registrar in Radiology
University Hospitals of Leicester NHS Trust
Leicester, UK

Anthony Dux
Consultant Radiologist and Honorary Senior Lecturer
University Hospitals of Leicester NHS Trust
Leicester, UK

WILEY-BLACKWELL
A John Wiley & Sons, Ltd., Publication

Library of Congress Cataloging-in-Publication Data

Clarke, Christopher, 1986–
  Chest x-rays for medical students / Christopher Clarke, Anthony Dux.
       p. ; cm.
  Includes bibliographical references and index.
  ISBN-13: 978-0-4706-5619-8 (pbk. : alk. paper)
  ISBN-10: 0-470-65619-0 (pbk. : alk. paper)
  1. Chest–Radiography–Atlases.   I. Dux, Anthony.   II. Title.
  [DNLM: 1. Radiography, Thoracic–methods–Atlases.   2. Thoracic
Diseases–radiography–Atlases.   3. Thorax–pathology–Atlases. WF 17]
  RC941.C593 2011
  617.5'407572–dc22

                                    2011007203

A catalogue record for this book is available from the British Library.

Set in 10 on 13 pt Frutiger Light by Toppan Best-set Premedia Limited

Printed and bound in Singapore by Markono Print Media Pte Ltd

4   2017

Contents

Preface

The chest X-ray is a frequently requested hospital investigation and often junior doctors are the first to review and act on the radiographs. Medical students therefore need to learn how to interpret basic signs and pathology on a chest X-ray.

I started developing this book in my final year of medical school while on a three-week 'student-selected component' in radiology at the University of Leicester. I realised that there was a need for more chest X-ray teaching resources for students at Leicester Medical School, so I started producing a chest radiograph teaching booklet, and my supervising consultant was immediately interested in the project. We have since developed this book, which has taken two years to write, with much of my time spent annotating and editing hundreds of X-rays.

The most novel and exciting aspect of *Chest X-rays for Medical Students* is the way colour overlays are used to highlight the anatomy and pathology. This way of 'marking' the radiographs separates this book from others and makes it easy to appreciate the sign or pathology of interest. Generally, two radiographs are displayed side by side, with the radiograph on the right marked out in colour and the radiograph on the left unmarked for comparison. This makes it easy to compare them and identify the abnormality on the unmarked radiograph. Some signs and pathologies are more difficult to appreciate and I experimented with many different enhancement techniques until I found one that worked. The result of this was that I have ended up using a range of different techniques to show or enhance pathology in this book.

This book is not intended to be used as an encyclopaedic reference but as a colourful and informative teaching aid to help medical students, junior doctors and radiographers learn the basics of chest X-ray interpretation in a simplified, logical and systematic way. We do not use confusing terms such as 'coin lesion', 'sail sign' or 'veil sign', as they are often used inaccurately and there are better ways to describe such radiological appearances.

I hope that by the end of this workbook you have a system to use for analysing and presenting chest radiographs and know how to recognise the important common pathologies on a chest X-ray.

We are constantly improving and refining this teaching resource for future students so would appreciate any feedback or suggestions you may have. Please feel free to contact us with any ideas you have.

Finally, we hope that you enjoy using this book.

Christopher Clarke
Anthony Dux

Note: In the self-assessment section, any initials, ages and dates used are purely fictitious and are not related to the patient's X-ray in question.

Acknowledgements

First, we would like to thank the radiographers and staff at University Hospitals of Leicester NHS Trust without whose dedication and work none of this would have been possible. We would like to thank the University of Leicester for the use of its libraries and excellent audiovisual services. Special thanks go to Leicester Medical School, in particular to Dr David Heney and Professor Stewart Peterson for their advice, encouragement and help with printing sample pages for a student feedback focus group. Without their support we would not have been able to publish this book. Special thanks also go to the many students who attended the focus group and lectures and gave fantastic feedback.

Their suggestions and contributions shaped this book and were invaluable.

We would like to acknowledge our friends and colleagues who have read this workbook and made numerous suggestions and contributions. Thanks to George Booth for his excellent electromagnetic spectrum illustration. Thanks to the reviewers for their excellent feedback and advice, spotting errors that would otherwise have been missed. Thanks to Martin Davies and Karen Moore from Wiley-Blackwell for giving us the opportunity to see our work published, and to all those people who remain unnamed in this acknowledgement, we are very grateful for your participation.

Learning objectives checklist

Keep track of your learning by ticking the ❑ when you have covered the topic.

By the end of this workbook, students should:

❑ Have a basic understanding of the principle of X-rays and how the image is produced.

❑ Have a system to use for analysing (ABCDE) and presenting chest radiographs.

❑ Know how to recognise the following on a plain PA erect chest X-ray:

  ❑ Rotation

  ❑ Adequate inspiration

  ❑ Tracheal deviation

  ❑ Carinal angle

  ❑ Consolidation/Airspace shadowing

  ❑ Air bronchogram

  ❑ Right upper lobe collapse

  ❑ Middle lobe collapse

  ❑ Right lower lobe collapse

  ❑ Left upper lobe collapse

  ❑ Left lower lobe collapse

  ❑ Complete lung collapse

  ❑ Pneumonectomy

  ❑ Solitary mass lesion

  ❑ Multiple mass lesions

  ❑ Cavitating lung lesion

  ❑ Fibrosis

  ❑ Pneumothorax

  ❑ Tension pneumothorax

  ❑ Hydropneumothorax

  ❑ Pleural effusion

  ❑ Pulmonary oedema

  ❑ 'Bat's wing' pattern shadowing

  ❑ Septal lines

  ❑ Dextrocardia

  ❑ Cardiomegaly (enlarged heart)

  ❑ Left atrial enlargement

  ❑ Widened mediastinum

  ❑ Hilar enlargement

  ❑ Hiatus hernia

  ❑ Rib fractures and other bony abnormalities

  ❑ Air under the diaphragm (pneumoperitoneum)

  ❑ Subcutaneous emphysema/Surgical emphysema

  ❑ Mastectomy

  ❑ Foreign bodies and medical interventions

❑ Know the following common conditions and their radiological signs:

  ❑ Bronchial carcinoma

  ❑ Heart failure

  ❑ Pneumonia

  ❑ Chronic obstructive pulmonary disease (COPD)

  ❑ Tuberculosis (TB)

  ❑ Asbestos-related lung disease:

    ❑ Benign pleural disease

    ❑ Asbestosis

    ❑ Malignant mesothelioma

About X-rays

What are X-rays?

X-rays are a form of **ionising radiation**. They are part of the electromagnetic spectrum and have sufficient energy to cause ionisation. They contain more energy than ultraviolet (UV) waves but less energy than gamma rays.

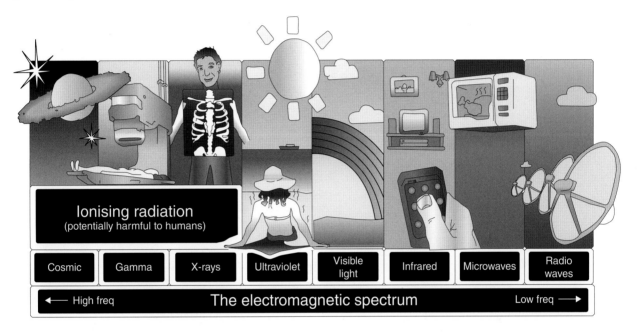

Figure 1 The electromagnetic spectrum.

Radiation: is the transfer of energy in the form of particles or waves.

Ionising radiation: is radiation with sufficient energy to cause ionisation, which is a process whereby radiation removes an outer-shell electron from an atom. Thus ionising radiation is able to cause changes on a molecular level in biologically important molecules (e.g. DNA).

Uses of ionising radiation: include conventional X-rays (plain film), contrast studies, computed tomography (CT), nuclear medicine and positron emission tomography (PET).

How are X-rays produced?

X-rays are produced by focusing a high-energy beam of electrons onto a tungsten target. If the electron has enough energy it can knock out another electron from the inner shell of a tungsten atom. As a result, electrons from higher energy levels then fill up this vacancy and X-rays are emitted. This process of producing X-rays is extremely inefficient (~0.1%), so most of the energy in the beam of electrons is wasted as heat. This is why X-ray tubes need to have advanced cooling mechanisms. The X-rays produced then pass through the patient and onto a detector mechanism, which produces an image.

Chest X-rays for Medical Students, First Edition. Christopher Clarke, Anthony Dux.
© 2011 John Wiley & Sons, Ltd. Published 2011 by Blackwell Publishing Ltd.

The resulting image on the X-ray film

Main points:

1. The resulting image on the X-ray film is a **two-dimensional (2D) representation of a three-dimensional (3D) structure**.

2. While passing through a patient the X-ray beam is absorbed in proportion to the cube of the atomic number of the various tissues through which it passes. By convention, the greater the amount of radiation hitting a detector, the darker the image will be. Therefore the less 'dense' a material is, the more X-rays get through and the darker the film will be. Conversely the more 'dense' a material is, the more X-rays are absorbed and the film appears whiter. **Materials of low 'density' appear darker than materials of high 'density'.**

3. **Structures can only be seen if there is sufficient contrast with surrounding tissues** (contrast is the difference in absorption between one tissue and another).

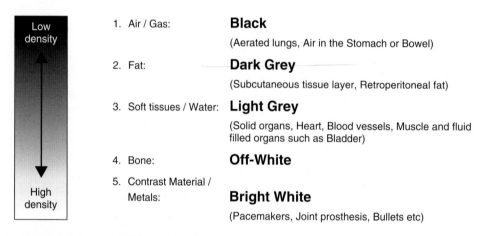

Figure 2 The spectrum of tissues of different densities as seen on a conventional radiograph.

How are X-ray images (radiographs) stored?

In some hospitals radiographs are printed onto X-ray film, but most now use a computer-based digital film storage system for storing X-ray images, thereby eliminating the need for film.

This system is known as **PACS** (**P**icture **A**rchiving and **C**ommunication **S**ystem). Doctors and other healthcare professionals are able to view the images (radiographs) on a computer screen, making it easy to manipulate the image (e.g. changing the contrast, zooming in/out, etc).

The advantages are ease of access, cost saving and no more lost films. The disadvantages are the initial cost and the risk of a system failure, which could be potentially catastrophic.

Hazards and precautions

Radiation hazards

Radiation hazards occur as a result of damage to cells by radiation. Actively dividing cells (i.e. bone marrow, lymph glands and gonads) are particularly sensitive. Damage takes many forms, including cell death, mitotic inhibition and chromosome/genetic damage leading to mutations.

The nature and degree of cell damage vary according to:
- radiation dose and dose rate
- volume of tissue irradiated
- type of radiation (alpha particles, X-rays, neutrons, etc).

IRMER 2000

Introduced in 2000, the Ionising Radiation (Medical Exposure) Regulations 2000 lay down the basic measures for radiation protection for patients. They refer to three main people involved in protecting the patient.

1. The **referrer** (a doctor or other accredited health professional [e.g. emergency nurse practitioner] requesting the exposure):
   - must provide adequate and relevant clinical information to enable the practitioner to justify the exposure.
2. The **practitioner** (usually a radiologist, who justifies the exposure):
   - decides on the appropriate imaging and justifies any exposure to radiation on a case-by-case basis. **Potential benefit must outweigh the risk to the patient** (e.g. a CT head scan on a 1-year-old adds a 1/500 lifetime risk of cancer and increases the risk of cataract formation. The benefit of this scan must therefore outweigh these risks to the child).
3. The **operator** (usually a radiographer, who performs practical aspects):
   - ensures that the above two stages have been completed appropriately
   - keeps all justifiable exposure as low as reasonably possible by:
     i. minimising the number of X-ray films taken
     ii. focusing the X-ray beam on the area of interest
     iii. minimising the use of mobile X-ray and using ultrasound or magnetic resonance imaging (MRI) if possible.

In women of reproductive age

- Minimise radiation exposure of abdomen and pelvis.
- Ask any woman of reproductive age if they could be pregnant and avoid radiation exposure in pregnant women. The most critical period is around 3–4 months gestation, when fetal organogenesis is taking place, and the fetus is considered to be radiosensitive. X-rays of the abdomen and pelvis should be delayed (if possible) to a time when fetal sensitivity is reduced (i.e. post-24 weeks gestation, or ideally until the baby is born).
- Exposure to remote areas (chest, skull and limbs) may be undertaken with minimal fetal exposure at any time during pregnancy.

Chest X-rays for Medical Students, First Edition. Christopher Clarke, Anthony Dux.
© 2011 John Wiley & Sons, Ltd. Published 2011 by Blackwell Publishing Ltd.

Chest X-ray (CXR) views

The standard view is a **PA (posterior–anterior) erect** chest X-ray. All chest X-rays are taken **PA erect** unless otherwise stated. You should always assume that a chest radiograph is PA erect, unless it has **AP** or **supine** printed on it.

PA erect CXR

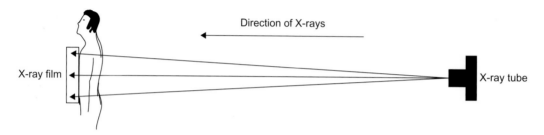

Figure 3 Posterior–anterior (PA) erect chest X-ray.

The patient stands with their anterior chest well up against an X-ray film. The X-ray tube is placed optimally 6 ft behind the patient so the X-rays pass in the posterior–anterior direction. The patient takes a deep breath and holds it during the X-ray to ensure there is adequate inspiration.

Reasons for performing the film PA
1. **Accurate assessment of the cardiac size due to minimal magnification.**
2. **The scapulae can be rotated out of the way.**

Reasons for performing the film erect:
1. **Gas passes upwards**: pneumothorax and free air underneath the diaphragm are more easily diagnosed.
2. **Fluid passes downwards**: pleural effusion is more easily diagnosed.
3. **Physiological representation of blood vessels and lungs** (if it were taken in the supine position, the mediastinal veins and upper lobe vessels may be more distended than normal, leading to misinterpretation).

Other views

- **AP (anterior–posterior)/supine CXR** is performed when the patient is too ill to stand (e.g. Intensive Care Unit or A&E Resuscitation). The X-ray tube is placed in front of the patient and the X-rays pass in the anterior–posterior direction. The major disadvantage of AP/supine films when compared with PA films is that the **mediastinum and cardiac size will appear wider** on an AP/supine film due to venous distension and magnification. Therefore you **SHOULD NOT** comment on the cardiac or mediastinal size on an AP/supine film.
- **Lateral CXR** is used to give further views of the lungs and heart, and more details on the anatomical location of lesions. It is rarely performed now as CT gives more information.
- **Expiratory PA erect CXR** is used rarely for helping to detect a suspected pneumothorax or suspected bronchial obstruction with air trapping.

Chest X-rays for Medical Students, First Edition. Christopher Clarke, Anthony Dux.
© 2011 John Wiley & Sons, Ltd. Published 2011 by Blackwell Publishing Ltd.

Normal anatomy on a PA chest X-ray

The following seven PA chest radiographs are identical and show the normal chest anatomy.

Normal anatomy 1 (Figure 4)

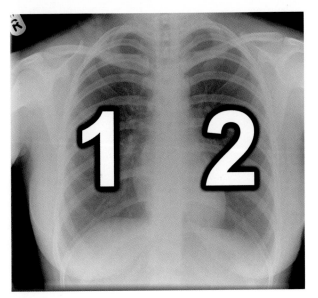

Remember, as you look at a chest X-ray, the left side of the radiograph is the patient's right side, and the right side of the radiograph is the patient's left side.

1. The patient's **RIGHT SIDE**.
2. The patient's **LEFT SIDE**.

Note: A good way to remember this is to imagine that the patient is always facing towards you. This is true for both PA and AP films.

Figure 4

Normal anatomy 2 (Figure 5)

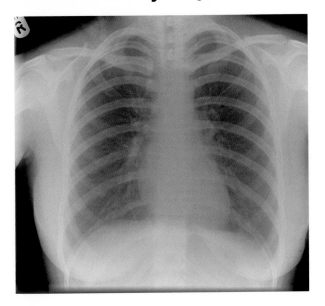

The mediastinum

The mediastinum is the central compartment of the thoracic cavity. It is marked in orange.

It contains the heart, the great vessels, oesophagus, trachea, phrenic nerve, vagus nerve, sympathetic chain, thoracic duct, thymus and central lymph nodes (including hilar lymph nodes).

Figure 5

Chest X-rays for Medical Students, First Edition. Christopher Clarke, Anthony Dux.
© 2011 John Wiley & Sons, Ltd. Published 2011 by Blackwell Publishing Ltd.

Normal anatomy 3 (Figure 6)

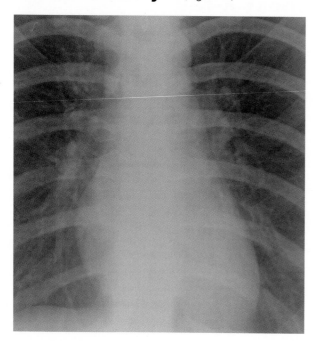 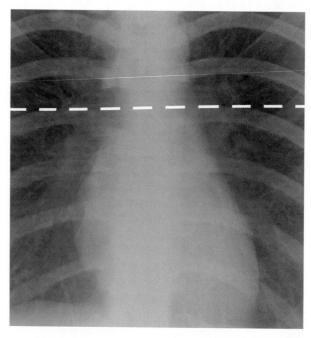

Figure 6

Normal pulmonary vascular patterns
The normal lung vascular pattern has the following features:
- **arteries** and **veins** branching **vertically** to upper and lower lobes
- **the upper lobe vessels have a smaller diameter than the lower lobe vessels** on an **erect CXR**.

The two images above are identical and show mediastinum and pulmonary vascular markings of a normal chest radiograph. The white dotted line is the level at which the pulmonary vessels enter and leave the lungs. The vessels are marked in red and you can see that the vessels branching upwards (the vessels above the white dotted line) are generally smaller than the vessels branching downwards (the vessels below the white dotted line). This is due to the effects of gravity.

Note: The opposite can occur in pulmonary venous hypertension, i.e. the vessels branching upwards become larger than the vessels branching downwards.

Normal anatomy 4 (Figure 7)

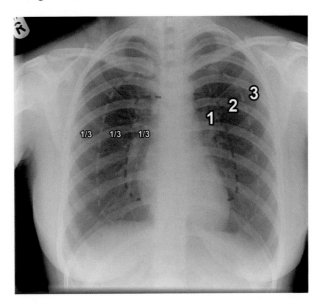

Figure 7

Normal lung markings

The lung markings are actually blood vessels in the lungs. They are visible on a chest radiograph as the X-rays are absorbed by the iron in the blood. If each lung is divided into thirds, from the inside to the outside, you can appreciate how the normal lung markings change:

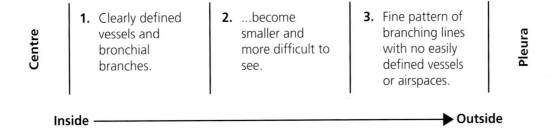

Centre	1. Clearly defined vessels and bronchial branches.	2. ...become smaller and more difficult to see.	3. Fine pattern of branching lines with no easily defined vessels or airspaces.	Pleura

Inside ⟶ Outside

Normal anatomy 5 (Figure 8)

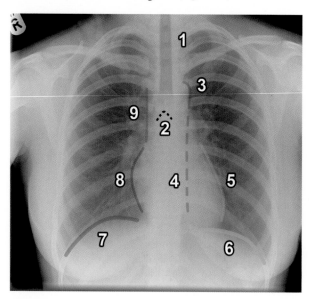

Figure 8

1. **Trachea** (light blue)
2. **Carina – spinal level T5** (black dotted line)
3. **Aortic arch/knuckle** (green)
4. **Descending thoracic aorta** (green dotted line)
5. **Left ventricle** (yellow)
6. **Left hemidiaphragm** (pink)
7. **Right hemidiaphragm** (purple)
8. **Right atrium** (red)
9. **Superior vena cava** (blue)

Note: The left ventricle forms the left heart border and the right atrium forms the right heart border. Neither the left atrium nor the right ventricle is visible on the normal chest radiograph. This is because the right ventricle lies anteriorly and the left atrium lies posteriorly, and they therefore have no definable border on a chest X-ray.

Normal anatomy 6 (Figure 9)

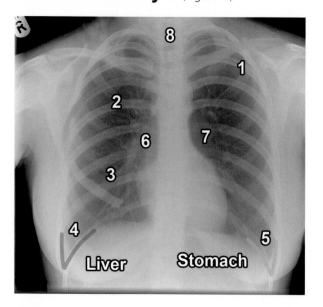

Figure 9

1. **Clavicle** (green)
2. **Posterior rib** (red)
3. **Anterior rib** (yellow)
4. **Right costophrenic angle** (purple)
5. **Left costophrenic angle** (pink)
6. **Right hilum** (containing the right hilar lymph nodes) (light blue)
7. **Left hilum** (containing the left hilar lymph nodes) (blue)
8. **Lung apex** (*pl.* apices) (orange)

Normal anatomy 7 (Figure 10)

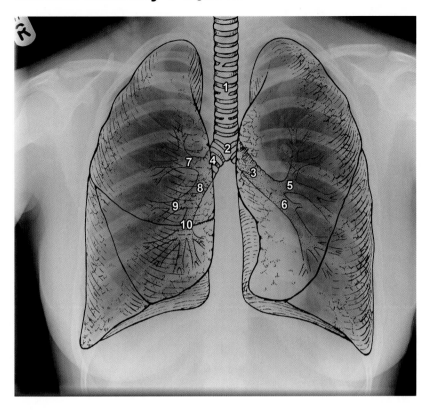

Figure 10

1. **Trachea**
2. **Carina** – spinal level T5
3. **Left mainstem bronchus**
4. **Right mainstem bronchus**
5. **Left upper lobe bronchus**
6. **Left lower lobe bronchus**
7. **Right upper lobe bronchus**
8. **Intermediate bronchus**
9. **Middle lobe bronchus**
10. **Right lower lobe bronchus**

Normal anatomy 8 (Figure 11)

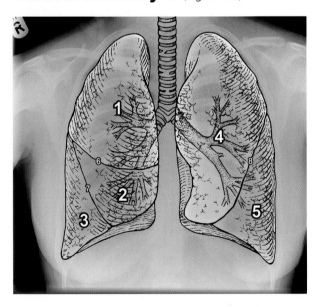

Figure 11

1. **Right upper lobe** (pink)
2. **Middle lobe** (purple)
3. **Right lower lobe** (blue)
4. **Left upper lobe** (pink)
5. **Left lower lobe** (blue)
6. **Horizontal** (lesser) **fissure**
7. **Right oblique fissure**
8. **Left oblique fissure**

The right upper lobe is separated from the middle lobe by the **horizontal** (lesser) **fissure**.

The middle lobe is separated from the right lower lobe by the **right oblique fissure**.

The left upper lobe is separated from the left lower lobe by the **left oblique fissure**.

Note: Remember the anatomy of the lungs. There is one middle lobe and it is in the right lung. As it is only found on the right side there is no need to describe it as 'right middle lobe'. You should simply call it the 'middle lobe'.

Presenting a chest radiograph

Be systematic

You should present a chest radiograph in a systematic way to ensure you cover all areas and do not miss anything important. This is how you should present.

1. Give the **type** of radiograph and **projection**.
2. Give the patient's name.
3. Give the date the X-ray was taken.
4. Briefly assess the film quality to ensure it is adequate.
5. Run through the ABCDE of chest X-rays.
6. Give a short summary at the end.

e.g. *'This is a **PA chest radiograph** of John Smith, taken on the 1ˢᵗ January 2012'*

See sections on 'Film quality' and 'The ABCDE of chest X-rays'

Remember always to describe what you are seeing. A good way to think about this is to **imagine you are describing the X-ray to a blind person**. If you see something you must say **where it is anatomically** and **what it looks like**.

There are 18 examples of describing a CXR on page 108.

Example of presenting a normal chest X-ray

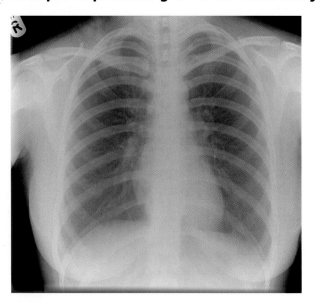

'This is a PA chest radiograph of Mrs LA, taken on the 24th of December 2011.'

'The film is not rotated and there is adequate inspiration.'

A: 'The trachea is central.'

B: 'The lungs are uniformly expanded and the lung fields are clear.'

C: 'The heart size is normal. There is no mediastinal shift. The mediastinal contours and hila appear normal.'

D: 'There is no fracture or bony abnormality.'

E: 'There is no evidence of air under the diaphragm, surgical emphysema or any foreign body.'

'In summary, this is a normal chest radiograph.'

Figure 12 Name: Mrs LA, age 50. Date taken: 24/12/2011.

Chest X-rays for Medical Students, First Edition. Christopher Clarke, Anthony Dux.
© 2011 John Wiley & Sons, Ltd. Published 2011 by Blackwell Publishing Ltd.

Film quality

Before you think about the possible abnormalities on a chest radiograph, you must first assess the technical quality of the film to ensure the image is adequate. There are two things you need to look for.

1. Rotation.
2. Adequate inspiration:
    – adequate inspiration is important as if the inspiration is too shallow the heart may appear falsely enlarged, giving the false appearance of cardiomegaly. Also if the lungs are not adequately inflated, the vessels at the lung bases can look more prominent and give the false appearance of consolidation or collapse.

> **Note:** You may find that some doctors will also want you to comment on whether the exposure of the film is adequate. However, this is no longer necessary, as images that are over- or under-exposed are terminated almost straight away by the radiographer and taken again. Also with a computer X-ray viewer, you can change the contrast and brightness with the mouse to compensate for poor exposure.

Rotation

Look at the spinous processes of the upper thoracic vertebrae. If the patient is not rotated they should lie midway between the medial ends of the clavicles. If the patient is rotated the spinous processes of the upper thoracic vertebrae will not lie midway between the medial ends of the clavicles but will be deviated to either the left or right.

- **Patient is rotated to the left:** the medial ends of the clavicles will be deviated to the left of the spinous processes of the upper thoracic vertebrae.
- **Patient is rotated to the right:** the medial ends of the clavicles will be deviated to the right of the spinous processes of the upper thoracic vertebrae.

> **Note:** This rule applies to both PA and AP films.

It is important to assess rotation as a rotated film can make the heart and mediastinum look larger or smaller than they actually are.

E.g. if normal: 'The patient is not rotated'

Normal example

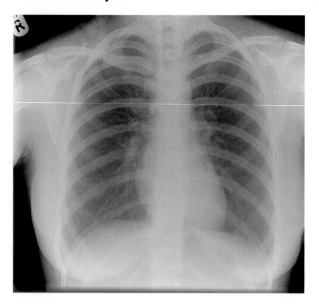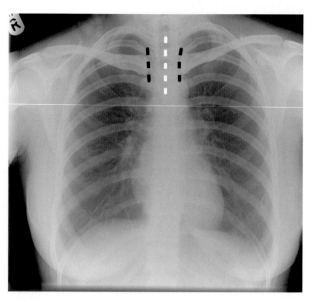

Figure 13 Two normal, identical chest radiographs. The spinous processes of the upper thoracic vertebrae lie midway between the medial ends of the clavicles, therefore this radiograph is *not* rotated. The right radiograph shows the clavicles marked in yellow. The medial ends of the clavicles are marked with a black dotted line. The position of the spinous processes is marked with a white dotted line.

Rotated example

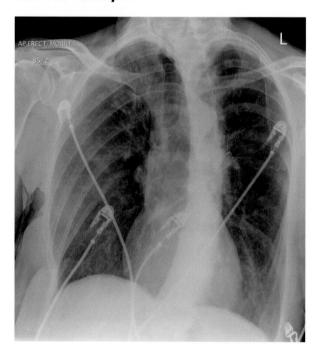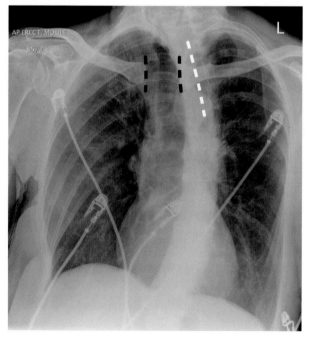

Figure 14 Two identical chest radiographs showing a patient rotated to the right. The medial ends of the clavicles are deviated to the right of the spinous processes of the upper thoracic vertebrae, therefore this radiograph is rotated to the right. The right radiograph shows the clavicles marked in yellow. The medial ends of the clavicles are marked with a black dotted line. The position of the spinous processes is marked with a white dotted line.

Adequate inspiration

If the hemidiaphragms lie at the level of the sixth anterior rib or below, then the inspiration is adequate. Alternatively, if there are eight or nine posterior ribs visible in the lung fields, this also indicates adequate inspiration.

E.g. if normal: 'There is adequate inspiration'

Example of adequate inspiration

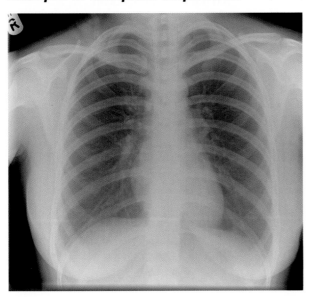
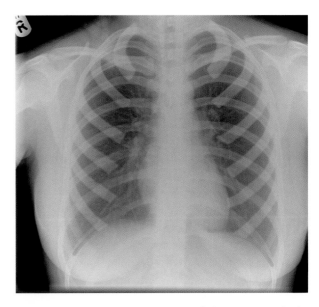

Figure 15 Two normal, identical chest radiographs. The right radiograph shows the anterior parts of ribs 1 to 6 marked in yellow. The left and right hemidiaphragm are marked in orange. Note how the diaphragm has a normal domed shape and not flattened.

If the lungs are under-inflated then there will be five or fewer anterior ribs (or seven or fewer posterior ribs) visible overlying the lung fields.

Example of inadequate inspiration

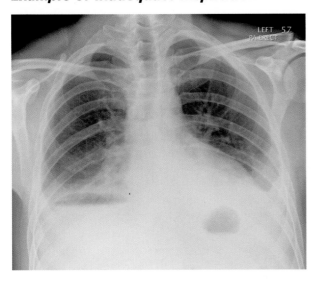
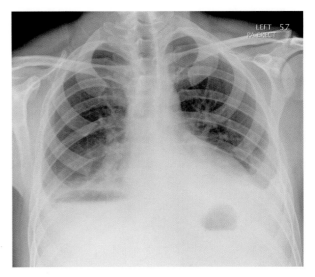

Figure 16 Two identical chest radiographs showing lung under-inflation. Notice how the lung volume has markedly decreased. There is the false appearance of cardiomegaly. The right radiograph shows the anterior parts of ribs 1 to 4 marked in yellow and the flattened hemidiaphragms marked in orange. (You can also see: air under the right hemidiaphragm.)

Overview of the ABCDE of chest X-rays

It is important to use a systematic approach when looking at a chest radiograph. The following ABC approach is easy to remember, so when it comes to your exams and you have a moment of panic after being asked to talk about a chest X-ray, you can stick to these basics even if you don't have a clue what's going on!

A is for Airway
- Look at the trachea, right and left mainstem bronchi and intermediate bronchus.

B is for Breathing
- Look to see if the lungs are uniformly expanded and compare the lung fields.
- Look around the edges of each lung.
- Look at the four silhouettes.

C is for Circulation
- Look at the cardiac size.
- Look at the great vessels (pulmonary vessels and aorta).
- Look at the mediastinum and hila.

D is for Disability
- Look for a fracture, especially of the ribs or shoulder girdle.

E is for Everything else
- Look for air under the diaphragm.
- Look at the edges for surgical emphysema.
- Look for the breast shadows.
- Look for foreign bodies and other 'unnatural presences'.

Chest X-rays for Medical Students, First Edition. Christopher Clarke, Anthony Dux.
© 2011 John Wiley & Sons, Ltd. Published 2011 by Blackwell Publishing Ltd.

The ABCDE of chest X-rays
What to look for in A – Airway

How to look

Start at the top and follow the **trachea (1)** inferiorly. It should be in the midline. It divides at the **carina (2)** to give off the **left mainstem bronchus (3)** and the **right mainstem bronchus (4)**.

On the left, the airway ends at the bifurcation of the left mainstem bronchus, where it splits into the **upper lobe bronchus (5)** and **lower lobe bronchus (6)**.

On the right, the right mainstem bronchus gives off the **upper lobe bronchus (7)** and continues inferiorly as the **intermediate bronchus (8)**. The airway ends at the bifurcation of the intermediate bronchus, where it splits into the **middle lobe bronchus (9)** and **lower lobe bronchus (10)**.

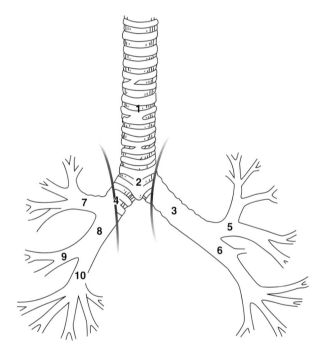

Figure 17 The airways of the lung.

What to look for

• Tracheal deviation	p. 21
• Carinal angle	p. 22

E.g. if normal: 'The trachea is central'

Chest X-rays for Medical Students, First Edition. Christopher Clarke, Anthony Dux.
© 2011 John Wiley & Sons, Ltd. Published 2011 by Blackwell Publishing Ltd.

What to look for in B – Breathing

How to look

The basic rule is that **black = air** and **white = no air**. There are five main things to look at.

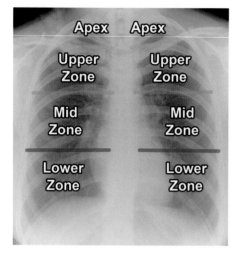

Figure 18 Zones of the lung.

1. Are the lungs **uniformly expanded**?
2. **Compare the lung fields** and look for white areas (shadows):
   – compare left apex with right apex
   – compare left upper zone with right upper zone
   – compare left mid zone with the right mid zone
   – compare the left lower zone with the right lower zone.
3. Look around the **edges** of each lung.
4. Look at the **costophrenic angles** (*see* p. 8)

5. Look for the **four silhouettes** (*see* Figure 19)

   i. Right heart border. Loss of the right heart border indicates a loss of air in the **middle lobe** (due to collapse or consolidation).

   ii. Left heart border. Loss of the left heart border indicates a loss of air in the **lingula** (the equivalent to the middle lobe in the left lung).

   iii. Right hemidiaphragm. ⎤ Loss of the clear diaphragmatic silhouette indicates there is loss of air
   iv. Left hemidiaphragm. ⎦ in the **lower lobe** (collapse or consolidation) or that there is something between the diaphragm and the lower lobe of the lung (e.g. fluid).

The four silhouettes

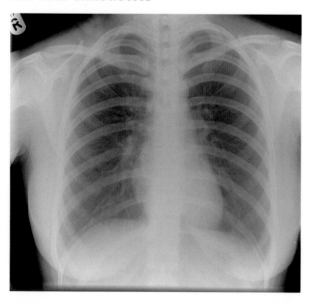
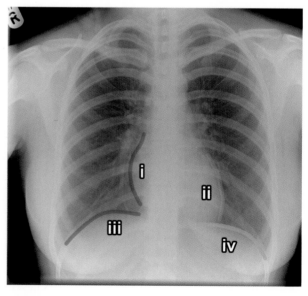

Figure 19 Two normal, identical chest radiographs. The four silhouettes are marked on the right radiograph. The right heart border is shown in red (i). The left heart border is shown in yellow (ii). The right hemidiaphragm is shown in purple (iii). The left hemidiaphragm is shown in pink (iv).

Chest X-rays for Medical Students, First Edition. Christopher Clarke, Anthony Dux.
© 2011 John Wiley & Sons, Ltd. Published 2011 by Blackwell Publishing Ltd.

What to look for

Chest X-rays do not show many specific diseases (e.g. pneumonia, bronchial carcinoma, etc.), only signs of pathology, which can give a clue to the underlying disease process. The following are a list of pathologies and signs that you should know.

E.g. if normal: 'The lungs are uniformly expanded and the lung fields are clear'

What to look for in C – Circulation

How to look

- Look at the **cardiac size**. The **width** of the heart should be no more than half the total width of the thorax.
- Look at the **great vessels** (**pulmonary vessels** and **aorta**).

The Latin for heart is 'cor' (as in cor pulmonale); therefore remember to look at the **'core'** of the X-ray.

- Look at the **mediastinum**, **both hila** and look for a **hiatus hernia.**

What to look for

E.g. if normal: 'The heart size is normal. There is no shift of mediastinum. The mediastinal contours and hila appear normal'

Chest X-rays for Medical Students, First Edition. Christopher Clarke, Anthony Dux.
© 2011 John Wiley & Sons, Ltd. Published 2011 by Blackwell Publishing Ltd.

What to look for in D – Disability

How to look
- Look for any **fracture** (#) or **bony abnormality** of the **ribs**. Don't forget to **rotate** the radiograph 90°.

> **Note:** This is because when you look at a radiograph normally, your eyes are trained to look at the anatomy of the lungs and heart, etc. However, rotating the image tricks your brain, and your eyes tend to focus on the more dense parts (ribs and other bones) making it easier to spot a fracture or bony abnormality.

- Step closer to the radiograph and **follow the edges** of each individual bone to look for fractures. Look for areas of **blackness** within each bone and **compare** the density of the bones on both sides. They should be the same.
- Repeat, looking for any fracture or bony abnormality of the **vertebrae**, **clavicles** or **shoulder girdle**.

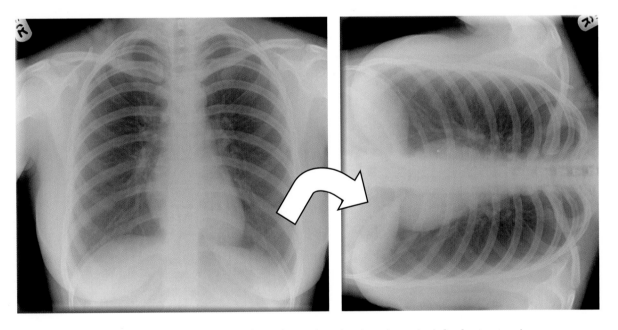

Figure 20 A normal chest radiograph. Rotating the radiograph makes it easier to look for fractures or bony abnormalities.

What to look for
- Rib fractures and other bony abnormalities   p. 80

E.g. if normal: 'I cannot see a fracture nor bony abnormality'

Chest X-rays for Medical Students, First Edition. Christopher Clarke, Anthony Dux.
© 2011 John Wiley & Sons, Ltd. Published 2011 by Blackwell Publishing Ltd.

What to look for in E – Everything else

How to look

- Look at the **hemidiaphragms** specifically for **air under the diaphragm**. Normally both hemidiaphragms peak in the centre and the right hemidiaphragm is higher than the left due to the position of the heart (not due to the liver). Other intra-abdominal pathologies you may see are areas of calcification under the right hemidiaphragm (gallstones) and dilated loops of bowel under the hemidiaphragms.
- Look at the **edges** of the body and all over the film for **surgical emphysema**.
- In a female patient look for the **breast shadows**. If one breast is smaller or missing, it could indicate a previous mastectomy (may explain secondary lung metastasis). Check axillae and lower neck for masses.
- Look for **foreign bodies** and '**other unnatural presences**'.

What to look for

- Air under the diaphragm (pneumoperitoneum)   p. 82
- Subcutaneous emphysema/Surgical emphysema   p. 84
- Mastectomy   p. 87
- Foreign bodies and medical interventions   p. 88

E.g. if normal: 'There is no evidence of air under the diaphragm, surgical emphysema nor any foreign body'

Chest X-rays for Medical Students, First Edition. Christopher Clarke, Anthony Dux.
© 2011 John Wiley & Sons, Ltd. Published 2011 by Blackwell Publishing Ltd.

Tracheal deviation

The trachea is considered to be deviated if a portion, anywhere along its length, is completely to the left or right of the midline (the midline being the centre of the vertebral column as indicated by the spinous processes).

> **Note:** Be sure to check that the film is not rotated, as a rotated film can give the impression of tracheal deviation when the trachea is actually central.

If you suspect that the trachea is deviated, look for a possible cause.
- **Deviated towards diseased side** (conditions that pull the trachea):
  - *lung collapse*
  - *pneumonectomy* (removal of a lung) or lobectomy (removal of just one lobe)
  - unilateral fibrosis
  - agenesis of lung (also called lung aplasia – complete absence of a whole lung and its bronchus).
- **Deviated away from diseased side** (conditions that push the trachea):
  - *tension pneumothorax*
  - *pleural effusion (large)*
  - mediastinal masses
  - para-tracheal masses.

(The most common causes of tracheal deviation are shown in **bold italic**.)

Most other processes (consolidation, non-tension pneumothorax, etc.) have little effect on tracheal deviation.

Example

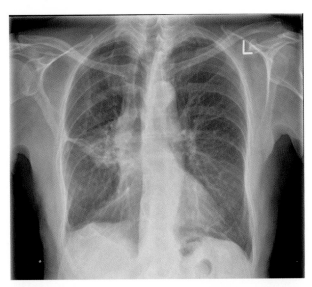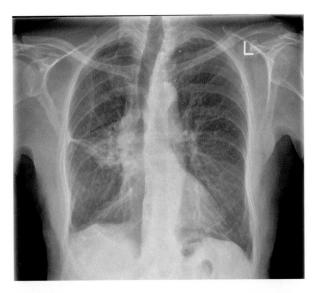

Figure 21 Two identical chest radiographs showing right tracheal deviation. The trachea is shown in blue on the right radiograph. (You can also see: mass lesion in the right lung and hilum, with resultant middle lobe collapse, pulling the trachea to the right.)

Carinal angle

The carinal angle is the **angle between** the **left mainstem bronchus** and the **right mainstem bronchus**. Normally the angle is between 40° and 100°. An **increase** in the **carinal angle** is an **indirect sign of pathology** in the heart, mediastinum or lungs, therefore if the carinal angle is greater than 100° look for a pathology that could be causing this.

It increases if there is something pushing from beneath the carina or if there is something pulling from above the right or left mainstem bronchus.

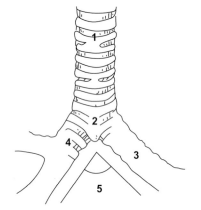

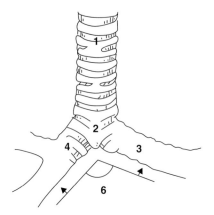

1. **Trachea**
2. **Carina** – spinal level T5
3. **Left mainstem bronchus**
4. **Right mainstem bronchus**
5. **Carinal angle**
6. **Widened carinal angle**

Figure 22 The carinal angle.

Figure 23 The carinal angle is widened, which could indicate pathology.

A widened carinal angle could indicate:
- **sub-carinal mass** (a mass below the carina, e.g. bronchial carcinoma, hiatal hernia)
- **left atrial enlargement**, **cardiomegaly** or a **pericardial effusion**
- **right or left upper lobe collapse** (pulling the mainstem bronchus upwards).

Example

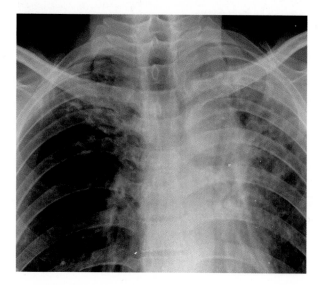

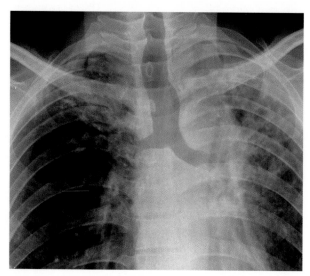

Figure 24 Two identical chest radiographs showing widening of the carinal angle. The carinal angle is greater than 100°. The right radiograph shows the trachea, right mainstem bronchus and left mainstem bronchus marked in blue.

Consolidation/Airspace shadowing

Consolidation (also known as airspace shadowing) is the **replacement of alveolar air** by **fluid, cells, pus** or **other material**. **Pneumonia** is by far the most common cause of consolidation. It is also sometimes seen in primary TB.

Features of consolidation on a chest radiograph
- **Patchy shadowing**: non-uniform shadowing and the border is not well demarcated.
- **Lobar or segmental density**: the density should correspond anatomically to a lobe or lung segment.
- **Air bronchogram** (*see* p. 27): the presence of an air bronchogram would confirm that the density (fluid/pus) was in the alveoli and not the larger airways. Bronchial breathing is the clinical equivalent of the air bronchogram.
- **No loss of lung volume**: lung volumes may actually increase in the early stages of consolidation. In later stages there can be a small loss of lung volume due to secretions obstructing airways; however, as a general rule, there is no significant loss of lung volume in consolidation.

> **Note:** Remember the clinical history. In the presence of a temperature and signs of infection, consolidation is by far the most likely abnormality. Also compare with previous X-rays – the presence of a similar abnormality on a previous X-ray should lead you to suspect fibrosis rather than consolidation.

Example 1

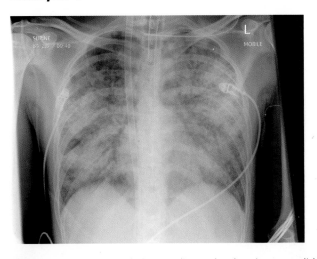
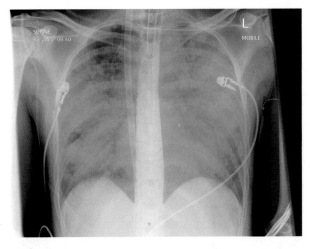

Figure 25 Two identical chest radiographs showing consolidation. There is consolidation in both lungs with moderate sparing of the apical segment of the right upper lobe (seen as darker than the rest). There is patchy airspace shadowing, no loss of lung volume and if you look carefully, you can see air bronchograms in both lungs. The right radiograph shows the consolidation marked in green. (You can also see: endotracheal tube in situ, nasogastric tube in situ, ECG leads and large cannula in superior vena cava.)

Example 2

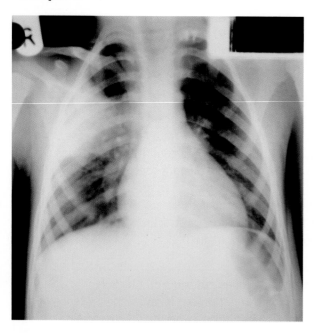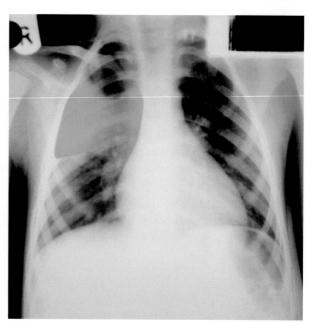

Figure 26 Two identical chest radiographs showing right upper lobe consolidation with sparing of the apical segment. The patchy airspace shadowing corresponds to the right upper lobe and there is no loss of lung volume. The right radiograph shows the consolidation marked in green.

Example 3

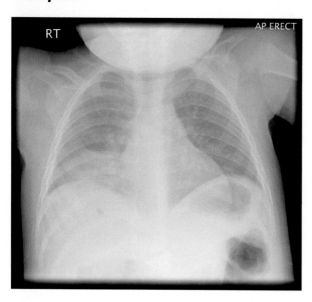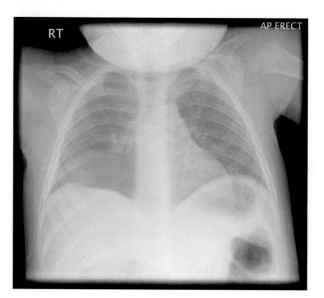

Figure 27 Two identical chest radiographs showing middle lobe consolidation. The patchy airspace shadowing corresponds to the middle lobe and there is no loss of lung volume. We know the consolidation is in the middle lobe as there is loss of the right heart border and the superior border is the horizontal fissure. The right radiograph shows the consolidation marked in green.

Example 4

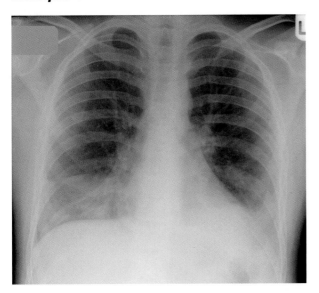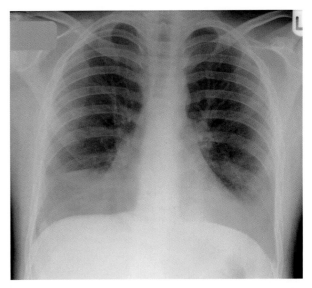

Figure 28 Two identical chest radiographs showing middle lobe and left lower lobe consolidation. The patchy airspace shadowing corresponds to the middle lobe and left lower lobe and there is no loss of lung volume. We know the consolidation is in the middle lobe as there is loss of the right heart border and the superior border is the horizontal fissure. We know the consolidation is in the left lower lobe as there is loss of definition of the left hemidiaphragm and the left heart border is still visible. The right radiograph shows the consolidation marked in green.

Example 5

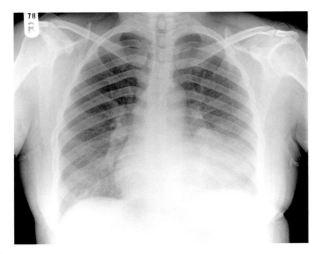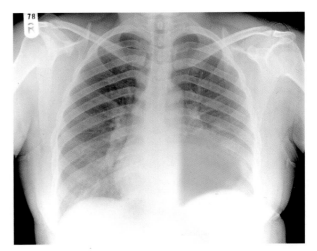

Figure 29 Two identical chest radiographs showing consolidation in the lingula. There is patchy airspace shadowing and no loss of lung volume. We know the consolidation is in the lingula as there is loss of the left heart border. The right radiograph shows the consolidation marked in green.

Example 6

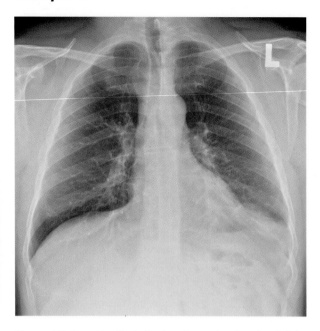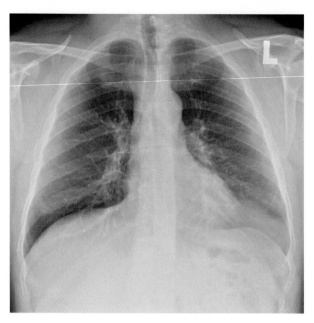

Figure 30 Two identical chest radiographs showing left lower lobe consolidation. The patchy airspace shadowing corresponds to the left lower lobe and there is no loss of lung volume. We know the consolidation is in the left lower lobe as there is loss of definition of the left hemidiaphragm. The right radiograph shows the consolidation marked in green.

Air bronchogram

An air bronchogram is the **radiographic appearance** of an **air-filled bronchus** that is surrounded by **fluid-filled** or **solid alveoli**.

- It can appear when there is **consolidation** (e.g. pneumonia), **collapse** or **pulmonary oedema** in the surrounding alveoli.
- Sometimes it is a good prognostic sign as it shows that secretions are able to exit from the consolidated region via the bronchus.

Note: The air bronchogram is the radiological equivalent of bronchial breathing on clinical examination.

B

Example 1

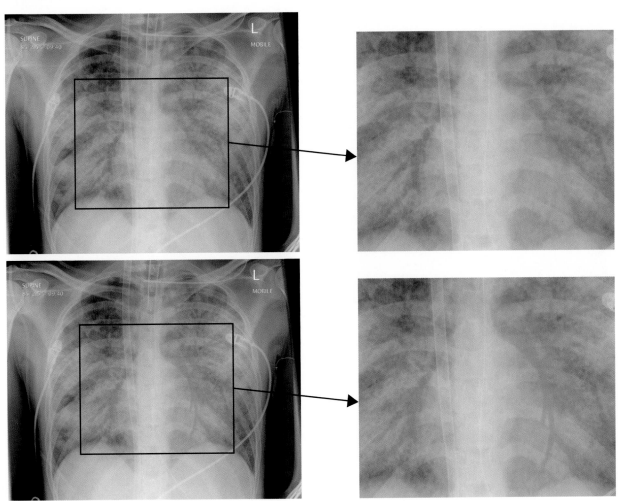

Figure 31 Two identical chest radiographs. This is an example of an air bronchogram caused by severe bilateral consolidation. The air bronchogram is marked in green on the inferior radiograph. (You can also see: endotracheal tube in situ, nasogastric tube in situ, ECG leads and large cannula in superior vena cava.)

B

Example 2

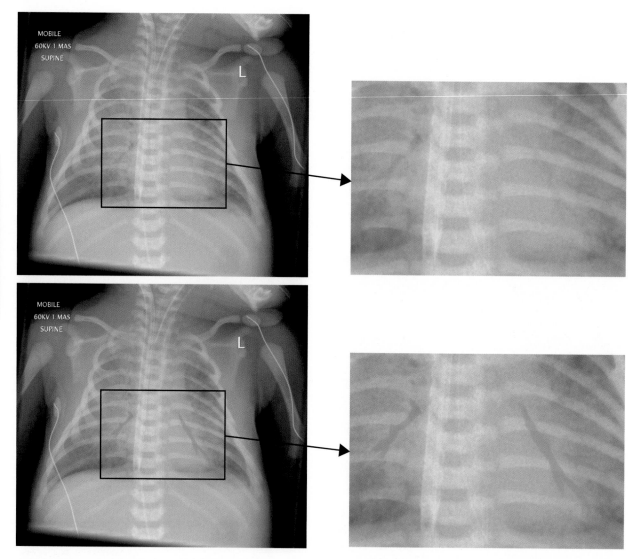

Figure 32 Two identical chest radiographs. This is an example of an air bronchogram caused by severe bilateral consolidation. The air bronchogram is marked in green on the inferior radiograph. (You can also see: endotracheal tube in situ, nasogastric tube in situ, ECG leads and large cannula in superior vena cava.)

Collapse (atelectasis) overview

Collapse is **failure of all or part of the lung to expand** due to **loss of air in the alveoli**.
- **Lobar collapse** refers to collapse of a particular lobe of the lung.
- **Lung collapse** refers to collapse of a whole lung.

General features of collapse on a chest radiograph include:
- An increase in **density**, representing lung devoid of air (whiteness).
- Signs indicating **decreased lung volume**, such as:
  - displacement of mediastinum/trachea towards the collapsed lung
  - elevation of the hemidiaphragm
  - compensatory over-inflation of adjacent lobes or opposite lung.

Note: When looking at a white lung, it is important to be thorough in looking for the possible features of collapse since the presence of collapse indicates possible serious pathology. Collapse is commonly found with consolidation (consolidation causing collapse). If this is so, it is referred to as collapse-consolidation.

Causes of collapse include:
- **Consolidation** (e.g. pneumonia).
- **Bronchial obstruction** by:
  - endobronchial tumour (a tumour invading one of the bronchi)
  - mucus plugging of major airways (asthma)
  - other tumours, lymphadenopathy or an aneurysm compressing the bronchi causing bronchial distortion
  - inhaled foreign body (e.g. peanut)
  - iatrogenic (endotracheal tube inserted too far).
- **External pulmonary compression (pleural effusion/collection** or **mass)**.
- Abnormalities of surfactant production (commonly occur with oxygen toxicity and acute respiratory distress syndrome).
- Inflammatory aetiology (e.g. tuberculosis or fungal infection).
- Lung fibrosis.

Specific signs of collapse of individual lobes are shown on the following pages.

B

Right upper lobe collapse

The right upper lobe collapses upwards.

Features of right upper lobe collapse on a chest radiograph

- Increased density in right upper zone.
- Horizontal fissure displaced upwards (pulled up by collapsed lobe).
- Loss of definition of right mediastinal margins.
- Elevation of right hilum (pulled up by collapsed lobe).
- Right tracheal deviation (collapsed lobe pulls trachea).
- The rest of the right lung looks blacker than the left lung (the middle lobe and right lower lobe over-inflate to compensate for the reduced volume in the hemithorax caused by the collapsed lobe).

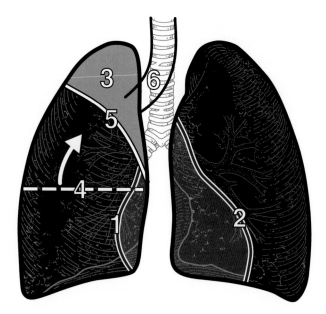

Figure 33 Diagrammatic representation of right upper lobe collapse. **1** Right heart border. **2** Left heart border. **3** Increased density in right upper zone. **4** Normal position of horizontal fissure. **5** Horizontal fissure displaced upwards. **6** Right tracheal deviation.

Example

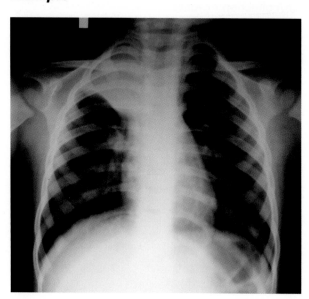
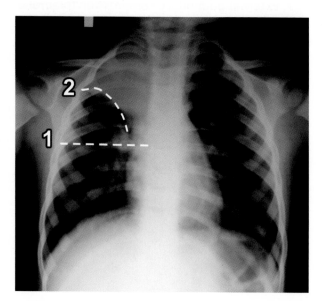

Figure 34 Two identical chest radiographs showing right upper lobe collapse. There is increased density of the right upper zone, elevation of the horizontal fissure and loss of definition of the upper right mediastinal margins. The right radiograph shows the collapsed right upper lobe in blue. The position of the horizontal fissure in a normal lung is shown with white dotted line **1** (often not visible on a radiograph). The abnormal position of the raised horizontal fissure in this radiograph is shown with white dotted line **2**.

Middle lobe collapse

The middle lobe collapses inwards.

Features of middle lobe collapse on a chest radiograph

- Increased density in right mid-zone.
- **Loss of the right heart border** (the collapsed lobe lies against the right heart border making it indistinct).
- Horizontal fissure displaced downwards (pulled down by collapsed lobe).
- The rest of the right lung looks blacker than the left lung (the right upper lobe and right lower lobe over-inflate to compensate for the reduced volume in the hemithorax caused by the collapsed lobe).

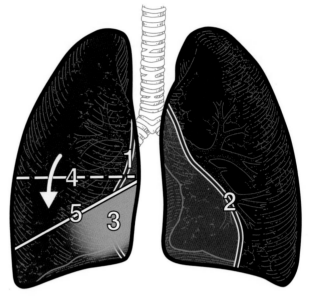

Figure 35 Diagrammatic representation of middle lobe collapse. **1** Right heart border. **2** Left heart border. **3** Increased density in right mid-zone. **4** Normal position of horizontal fissure. **5** Horizontal fissure displaced downwards.

Example

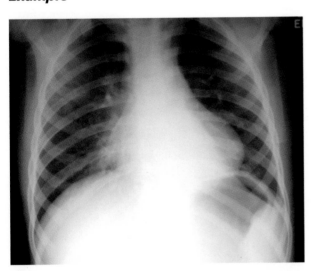
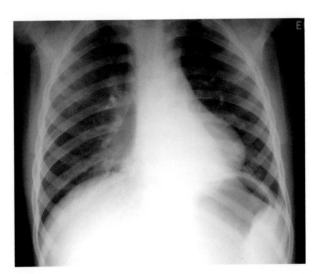

Figure 36 Two identical chest radiographs showing middle lobe collapse. There is an increased density in the right mid-zone and the right heart border is obscured. The right radiograph shows the collapsed middle lobe in blue. (You can also see: collapsed left lower lobe.)

Right lower lobe collapse

The right lower lobe collapses inferiorly and medially.

Features of right lower lobe collapse on a chest radiograph

- Triangular shadowing at the right base medially.
- Loss of definition of the right hemidiaphragm.
- Elevation of right hemidiaphragm (pulled up by collapsed lobe).
- Depression of right hilum (pulled down by collapsed lobe).
- **The right heart border is not obscured.**
- The rest of the right lung looks blacker than the left lung (the right upper lobe and middle lobe over-inflate to compensate for the reduced volume in the hemithorax caused by the collapsed lobe).

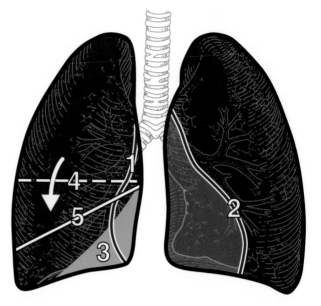

Figure 37 Diagrammatic representation of right lower lobe collapse. **1** Right heart border. **2** Left heart border. **3** Triangular shadowing at the right base medically. **4** Normal position of horizontal fissure. **5** Horizontal fissure displaced downwards.

Example 1

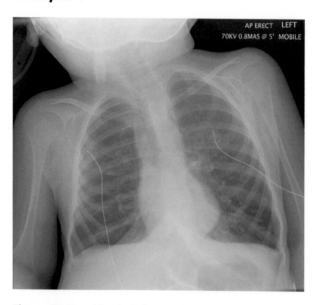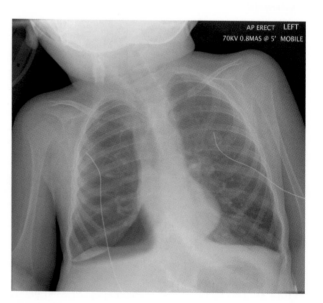

Figure 38 Two identical chest radiographs showing right lower lobe collapse. There is a triangular opacity at the right base medially and the heart border is not obscured. The right radiograph shows the collapsed right lower lobe in blue. (You can also see: ECG leads.)

Example 2

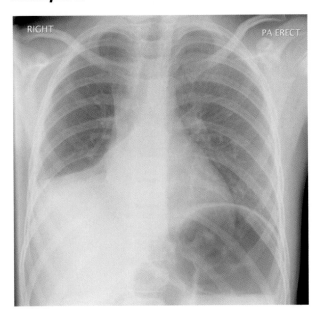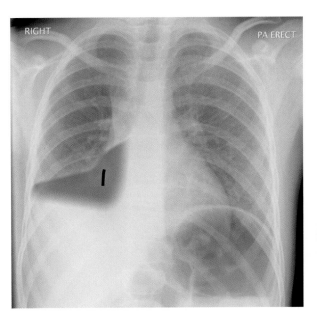

Figure 39 Two identical chest radiographs showing right lower lobe collapse. There is a triangular opacity at the right base medially, loss of definition of the hemidiaphragm and elevation of the right hemidiaphragm. If you look carefully you can still see the right heart border, therefore the collapse does not involve the middle lobe. The right radiograph shows the collapsed right lower lobe in blue and the right heart border is marked with a black line. (You can also see: large air bubble in the stomach with a fluid level – the gastric contents.)

Left upper lobe collapse

The left upper lobe collapses inwards and upwards.

Features of left upper lobe collapse on a chest radiograph

- Increased density of left upper zone.
- Upper zone 'veil-like' shadowing with no clear lower border.
- Loss of definition of left upper cardiac border and left mediastinal margin.
- Elevation of left hilum (pulled up by collapsed lobe).
- Left tracheal deviation (collapsed lobe pulls trachea).

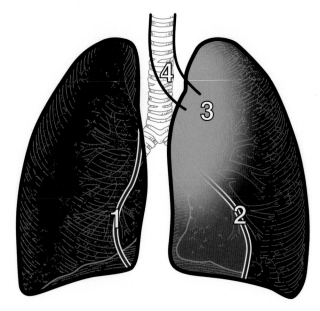

Figure 40 Diagrammatic representation of left upper lobe collapse. **1** Right heart border. **2** Left heart border. **3** Increased density of left upper zone with a 'veil-like' shadowing and no clear lower border. **4** Left tracheal deviation.

Example 1

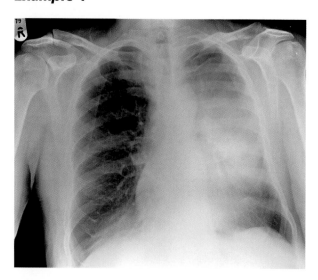 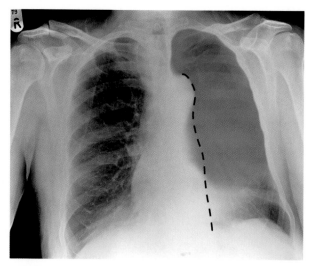

Figure 41 Two identical chest radiographs showing left upper lobe collapse. There is increased density of the left upper zone with no clear lower border, and a loss of definition of the left upper heart border and left mediastinal margin. You can, however, see the outline of the aortic arch and descending thoracic aorta (marked with a black dotted line). This indicates that there is air in the lung tissue directly adjacent to the aortic arch and descending thoracic aorta. The aorta lies in the posterior mediastinum so the aerated lung must be the posterior segment of the left upper lobe. This means that it must be the anterior segment of the left upper lobe that collapsed, i.e. the lingula. The right radiograph shows the collapsed left upper lobe in blue.

Example 2

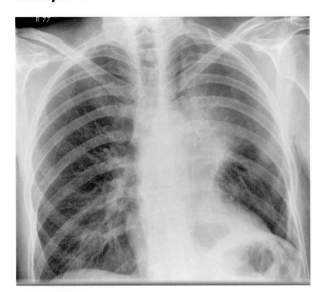 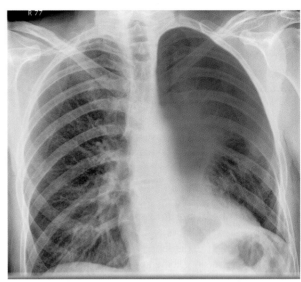

Figure 42 Two identical chest radiographs showing left upper lobe collapse. There is increased density of the left upper zone with no clear lower border and a loss of definition of the left mediastinal margin. The left heart border is still visible as the lingula remains inflated. The left apex and left upper zone still contain aerated lung because the left lower lobe has expanded up to the apex to fill the space left by the collapsed left upper lobe. This indicates that the collapse is likely chronic rather than acute as it takes time for the left lower lobe to expand to fill the space left by the collapsed upper lobe. The right radiograph shows the collapsed left upper lobe in blue.

Left lower lobe collapse

The left lower lobe collapses inferiorly and medially.

Features of left lower lobe collapse on a chest radiograph

- Triangular shadowing overlying the left heart medially (**'double heart'** shadow).
- Loss of definition of the medial part of the left hemidiaphragm.
- Elevation of the left hemidiaphragm (pulled up by collapsed lobe).
- Depression of left hilum (pulled down by collapsed lobe).
- **The left heart border is not obscured.**
- The rest of the left lung looks blacker than the right lung (the left upper lobe over-inflates to compensate for the reduced volume in the hemithorax caused by the collapsed lobe).

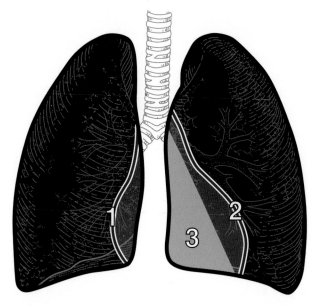

Figure 43 Diagrammatic representation of left lower lobe collapse. **1** Right heart border. **2** Left heart border. **3** Triangular shadowing overlying the left heart medially ('double heart' shadow).

Example 1

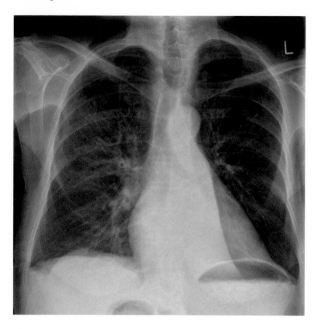
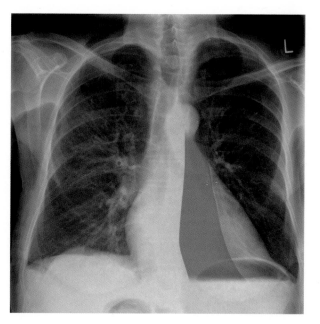

Figure 44 Two identical chest radiographs showing left lower lobe collapse. There is a triangular opacity behind the left heart shadow. The heart border is not obscured and there is decreased volume of the left lung. The right radiograph shows the collapsed left lower lobe in blue.

Example 2

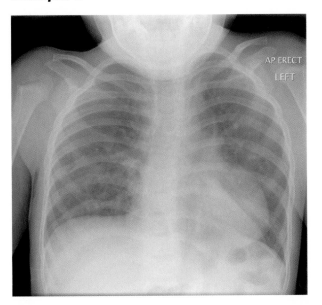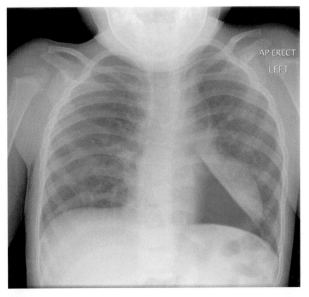

Figure 45 Two identical chest radiographs showing left lower lobe collapse. There is a triangular opacity behind the left heart shadow with loss of definition of the medial part of the left hemidiaphragm. The heart border is not obscured. The right radiograph shows the collapsed left lower lobe in blue.

Example 3

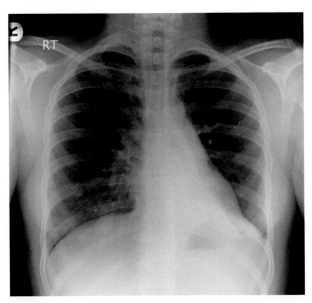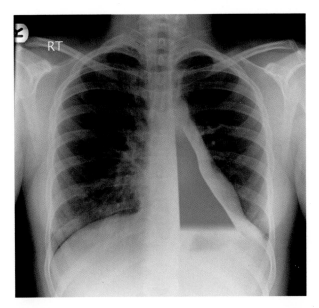

Figure 46 Two identical chest radiographs showing left lower lobe collapse. There is a triangular opacity behind the left heart shadow with loss of definition of the medial part of the left hemidiaphragm. The heart border is not obscured. The right radiograph shows the collapsed left lower lobe in blue.

Complete lung collapse

Example 1

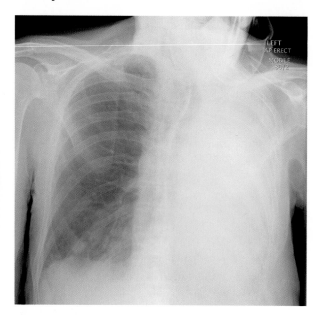

Figure 47 A chest radiograph showing complete collapse of the left lung. There is increased density throughout the entire left lung and signs of decreased lung volume, such as displacement of the mediastinum/hila towards the collapsed lung and left tracheal deviation.

Example 2

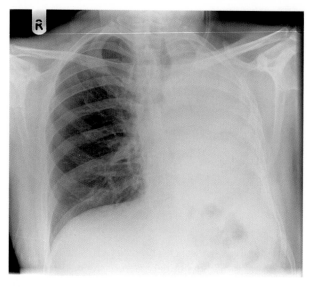

Figure 48 A chest radiograph showing complete collapse of the left lung. There is increased density throughout the entire left lung and signs of decreased lung volume, such as displacement of the mediastinum/hila towards the collapsed lung and left tracheal deviation.

Example 3

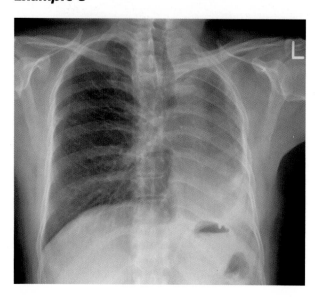
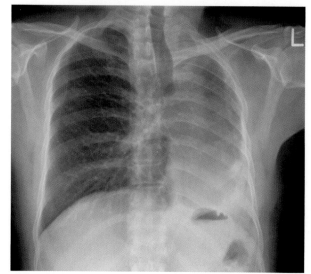

Figure 49 Two identical chest radiographs showing near complete collapse of the left lung (although there is still a minimal amount of air in the left upper lobe). There is increased density throughout the entire left lung and signs of decreased lung volume, such as displacement of the heart/mediastinum/hila towards the collapsed lung and left tracheal deviation. The deviated trachea is marked in blue.

Pneumonectomy

Pneumonectomy is an **operation to remove a whole lung**. You should know from the patient's history and your examination that the patient has had a previous pneumonectomy.

Radiological signs of a previous pneumonectomy
- **Diffuse haziness** and **loss of hemidiaphragm** where the lung has been removed.
- **Smaller hemithorax** where the lung has been removed and **hyperinflation of the opposite lung field** (appears darker).
- **Mediastinal/tracheal shift** towards the side with no lung.
- You may see **surgical clips** and/or evidence of **rib resection**.

Note: You cannot differentiate between a pneumonectomy and a complete lung collapse on a chest radiograph (unless you can see evidence of a previous thoracotomy) as they may both look the same.

Example 1

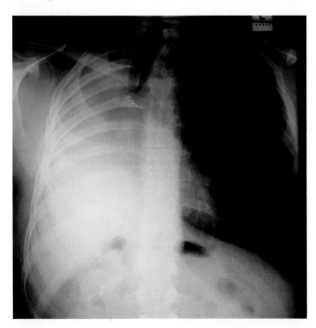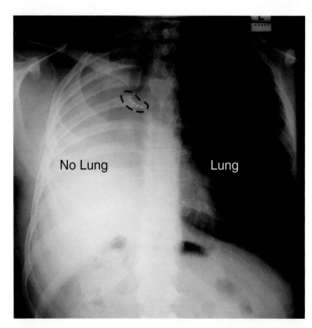

No Lung   Lung

Figure 50 Two identical chest radiographs showing evidence of a previous right pneumonectomy. There is diffuse haziness throughout the right hemithorax (debris and fluid). There is mediastinal shift towards the side of the operation (with associated tracheal deviation). If you look carefully, you can see sutures where the top of the right mainstem bronchus should be. The right radiograph shows the trachea marked in blue and the sutures highlighted in white, surrounded by a black dotted line.

B

Example 2

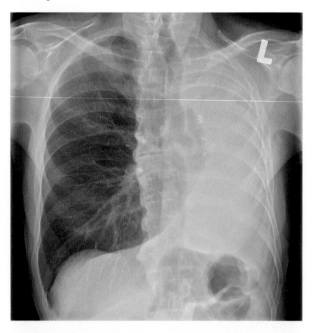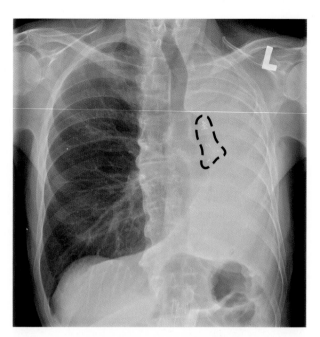

Figure 51 Two identical chest radiographs showing evidence of a previous left pneumonectomy. There is diffuse haziness throughout the left hemithorax (debris and fluid). There is mediastinal shift towards the side of the operation (with associated tracheal deviation). If you look carefully, you can see sutures in the left hemithorax. The right radiograph shows the trachea marked in blue and the sutures highlighted in white, surrounded by a black dotted line.

Example 3

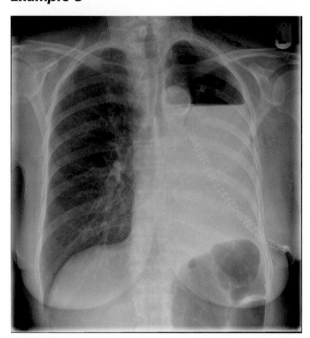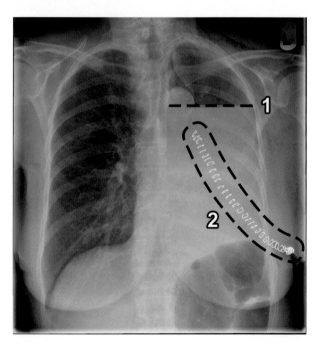

Figure 52 Two identical chest radiographs showing evidence of a previous left pneumonectomy. There is diffuse haziness (debris and fluid) in the inferior two thirds and air (pneumothorax) in the superior third of the left hemithorax. You can see a horizontal air-fluid level where the debris/fluid meets the air. There is a line of staples on the left side from the recent surgery. The right radiograph shows the pneumothorax marked in blue and the debris/fluid marked in green. The air-fluid level is shown with a black dotted line (**1**). The staples are highlighted in white and surrounded by a black dotted line (**2**).

Solitary mass lesion

A solitary mass lesion is a term used to describe a **discrete area** of **whiteness** situated within a lung field. It is not necessarily circular (it can be round, oval or irregular). The main worry is that it could be a carcinoma.

Radiological factors to assess

- **Size** – greater than 1 cm in diameter makes the lesion significant.
- **Margin** – irregular, lobulated or spiculated margin suggests malignancy.
- **Cavitation** (*see* p. 47) – both neoplasm and infection may cause cavitation.
- **Calcification** – would appear dense white (like bone). Rare in malignancy.
- **Compare with a previous CXR** – to assess growth.
- **Look for other solitary mass lesions**.

Differential diagnosis

1. **Neoplasm**
   - (a) **Primary bronchial carcinoma**
     - Evidence of rapid growth in a short time (multiple examinations).
     - Irregular, lobulated or spiculated margin.
     - No calcification.
   - (b) **Solitary metastasis**
     - Look for evidence of previous mastectomy – can give clue as to possible cause e.g. breast cancer.
2. **Benign mass lesion**
   - (a) **Intrapulmonary**, e.g. hamartoma (often contain calcium) and benign lung cysts.
   - (b) **Extrapulmonary**, e.g. neurofibromata.
3. **Infection**
   - (a) **Tuberculosis (TB)**
     - i. **Primary TB**
       - Peripheral lung mass/consolidation (Ghon focus).
       - Associated with enlarged hilar lymph nodes.
     - ii. **Tuberculoma** (remnants of previous TB infection)
       - Calcification common.
       - Well-defined margin.
       - Around 2 cm diameter.
       - Unchanged on serial CXR examinations.
   - (b) **Other infection**
     - Localised area of consolidation or abscess.
4. **Arteriovenous malformations**
   - Feeding arteries and draining veins may be seen.

B

B

Example 1

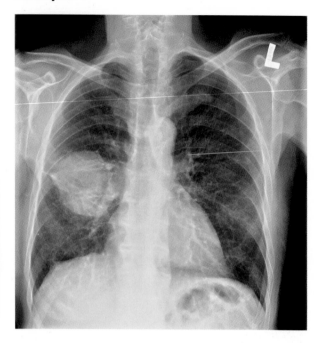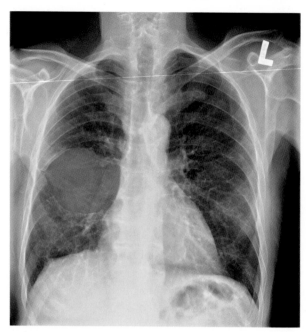

Figure 53 Two identical chest radiographs of a patient with a large mass lesion in the right upper lobe. The right radiograph shows the mass marked in red.

Example 2

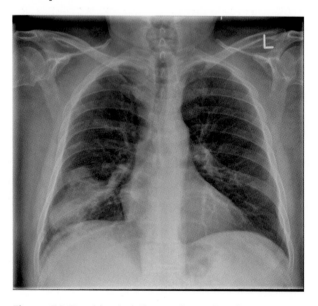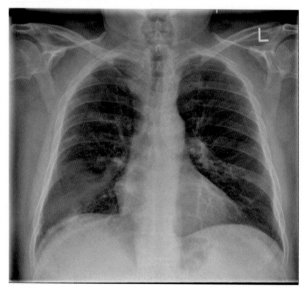

Figure 54 Two identical chest radiographs of a patient with a large mass lesion in the right lower lobe. The right radiograph shows the mass marked in red.

B

Example 3

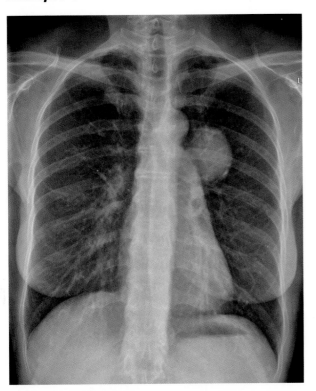
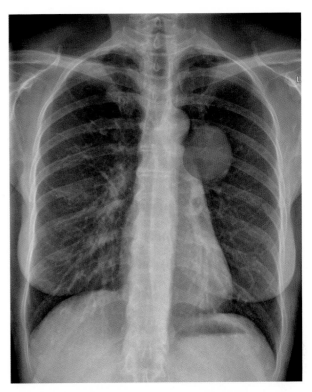

Figure 55 Two identical chest radiographs of a patient with a large mass lesion in the left lung. The right radiograph shows the mass marked in red.

Example 4

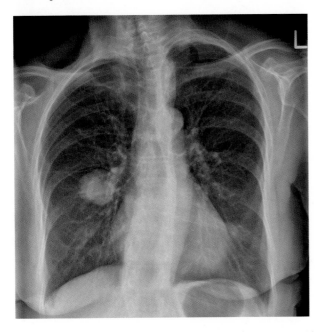
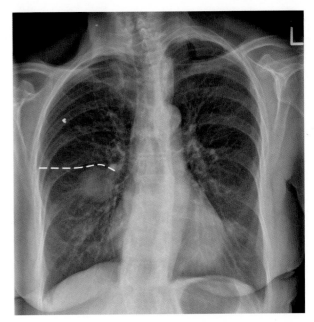

Figure 56 Two identical chest radiographs of a patient with a large mass lesion in the middle lobe. You know it is located in the middle lobe because if you look carefully you can see that the mass is pushing up the horizontal fissure, the fissure separating the right upper lobe and middle lobe. The right radiograph shows the mass marked in red. The white dotted line indicates the position of the horizontal fissure.

Multiple mass lesions

Differential diagnosis

1. **Metastasis**
   - Usually well defined.
   - Nodules of varying size.
   - Cavitation seen in squamous cell carcinomas, sarcomas and metastases from colonic primaries.
2. **Abscesses**
   - Cavitation with thick, irregular wall.

Rare and generally very small:

3. **Rheumatoid nodules**
4. **Wegener's granulomatosis**
   - Cavitation common.
5. **Multiple arteriovenous malformations**

Example 1

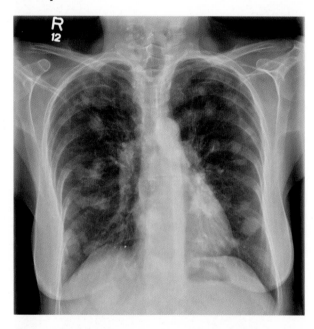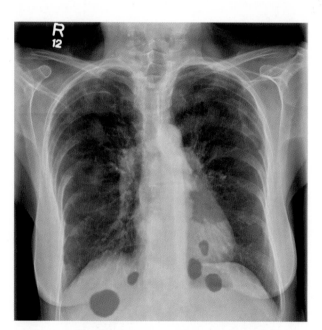

Figure 57 Two identical chest radiographs of a patient with multiple lung metastases throughout both lung fields. The right radiograph shows the metastases marked in red.

Example 2

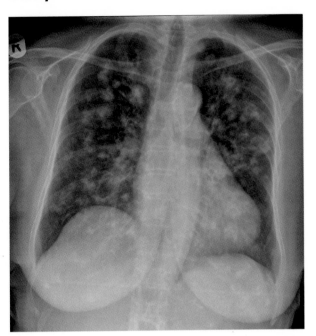
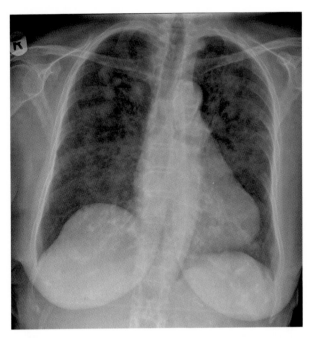

Figure 58 Two identical chest radiographs of a patient with multiple lung metastases throughout both lung fields. The right radiograph shows the metastases marked in red.

Example 3

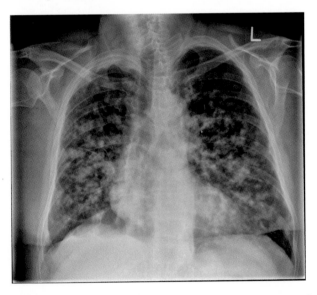
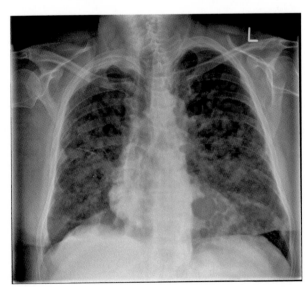

Figure 59 Two identical chest radiographs of a patient with multiple lung metastases throughout both lung fields. The right radiograph shows the metastases marked in red.

B

Example 4

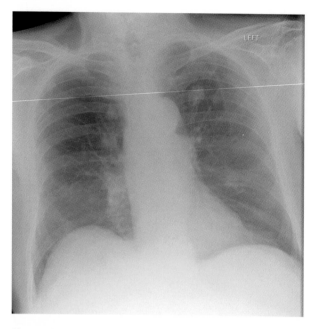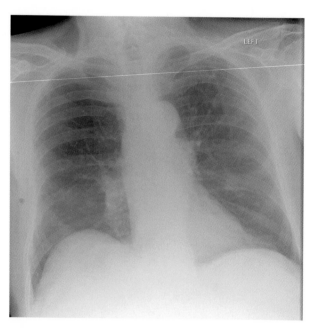

Figure 60 Two identical chest radiographs of a patient with multiple lung metastases. The right radiograph shows the metastases marked in red.

Example 5

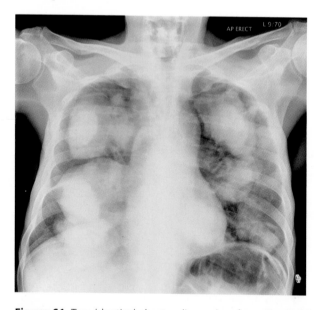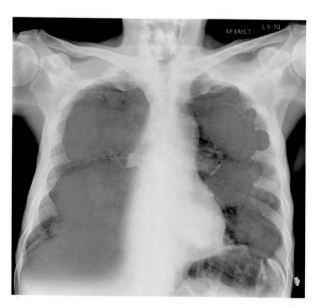

Figure 61 Two identical chest radiographs of a patient with multiple lung metastases. Interestingly, further investigation showed that these were from a massive untreated colonic carcinoma. The right radiograph shows the metastases marked in red.

Cavitating lung lesion

Solitary mass lesions may sometimes cavitate, causing a cavitating lung lesion. A cavitation is a **hole** in the lung with a **wall**, **lumen** and **contents**. A cavity is often easier to see from a distance so stepping away from the X-ray can help.

Causes of cavitation
- Abscess
- Neoplasm
- Cavitation around a pneumonia
- Fibrosis
- Rheumatoid nodules (rare)

Possible radiological signs
- **Centre** of the lesion is **darker** than the periphery as no blood passes through it.
- **Fluid level** present: look for a **horizontal line within the lesion**. There will be **whiteness (fluid) below** the line and **blackness (air) above** the line.
- Compare with old films (may be possible to see the cavity developing).

Note: If you see a cavitating lesion, look at the wall of the cavity. The thicker the wall, the more likely it is to be a neoplasm. Generally, if the wall is >5 mm thick, then it is more likely to be a neoplasm as opposed to an abscess.

Example 1

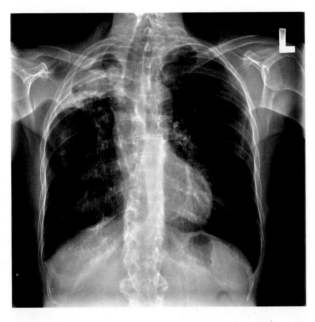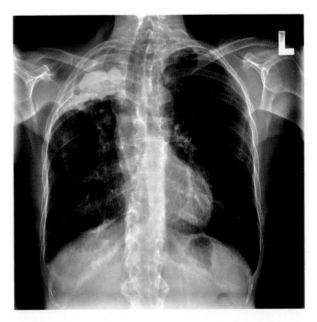

Figure 62 Two identical chest radiographs showing a cavitating lung lesion in the right upper lobe. Within the cavity is a fungal ball, which appears whiter than the rest of the cavity. The right radiograph shows the cavity in yellow. The fungal ball within the cavity is shown in light yellow.

B

Example 2

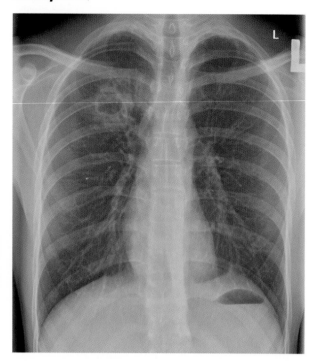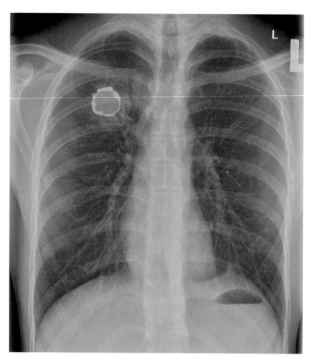

Figure 63 Two identical chest radiographs showing a cavitating lung lesion in the right upper zone. It is likely to be a mass lesion as there are no features of consolidation or fibrosis. The right radiograph shows the cavity in yellow. The wall of the cavity is shown in light yellow.

Example 3

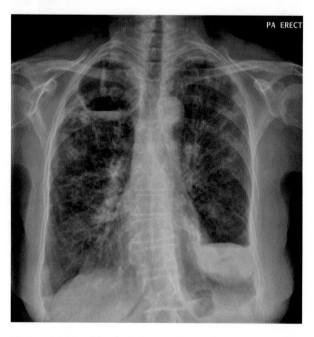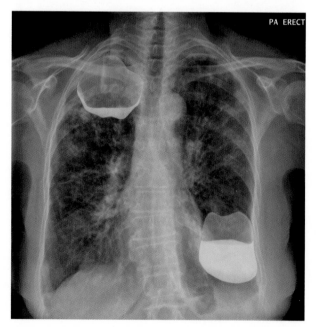

Figure 64 Two identical chest radiographs showing two cavitating lung lesions, one in the right upper lobe and the other in the left lower lobe. Both cavities are due to bullae, which have become infected. This explains the presence of both air and fluid. The right radiograph shows the cavities in yellow. The fluid within the cavities is shown in light yellow.

Fibrosis

Fibrosis is thickening and scarring of the **interstitium** (connective tissue) **of the lung**. The interstitium surrounds the bronchi, vessels and groups of alveoli. Interstitial fibrosis gives **reticulonodular** type **shadowing**.

Note: The main two processes affecting the interstitium are **accumulation of fluid** (occurring in pulmonary oedema or lymphangitis and giving rise to septal lines) and **inflammation leading to fibrosis** (giving rise to reticulonodular shadowing). On chest X-rays you need to differentiate reticulonodular shadowing from consolidation or pulmonary oedema (which are both far more common).

B

Causes of interstitial fibrosis
- Sarcoidosis
  - **S** Systemic sclerosis
  - **A** Asbestosis (p. 103)
  - **R** Rheumatoid
  - **C** Connective tissue disorders (SLE)
  - **O** Occupation (pneumoconiosis, extrinsic allergic alveolitis)
  - **I** Idiopathic pulmonary fibrosis (usual interstitial pneumonitis)
  - **D** Drugs (methotrexate, amiodarone, cyclophosphamide etc) + Chemicals
- Bronchiectasis
- TB (p. 98)
- Radiotherapy (usually following treatment for carcinoma of the breast)

i. Bird-fancier's lung
    (pigeon and budgie excretions)

ii. Farmer's lung
    (fungal spores from mouldy hay)

Radiological features of reticulonodular shadowing
- **Reticular shadowing:**
  - produced by **thickening** of the **lung interstitium** (connective tissue)
  - seen as a **fine** or **coarse branching linear pattern**. The heart loses its normal smooth outline and seems 'shaggy'.
- **Nodular shadowing:**
  - **small discrete opacities 1–5 mm in diameter**.

B

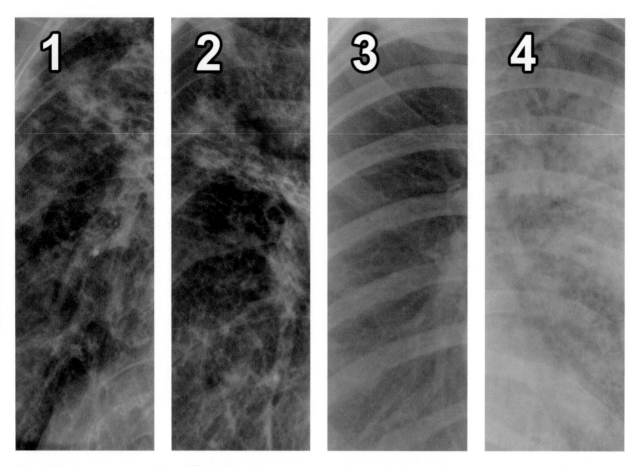

Figure 65 A comparison of four different X-ray appearances to help you appreciate the difference between fibrosis, normal lung and consolidation. **1 & 2** Reticulonodular type shadowing (fibrosis). **3** Normal lung appearance. **4** Consolidation.

Example 1

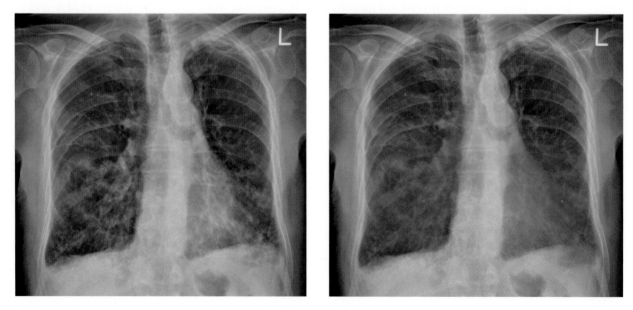

Figure 66 Two identical chest radiographs showing coarse mid- and lower zone fibrosis. There is reticulonodular type shadowing. The cause is unknown in this radiograph and would have to be determined by the patient's clinical history. The right radiograph shows the radiological features of fibrosis marked in purple.

Example 2

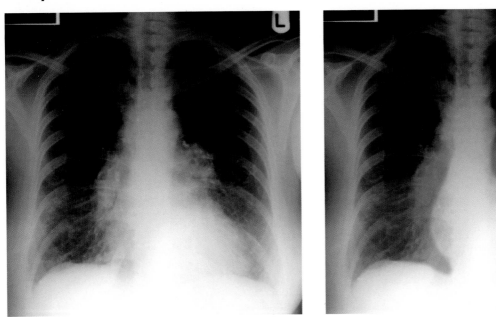

Figure 67 Two identical chest radiographs showing coarse mid- and lower zone fibrosis. There is reticular type shadowing. In this case the patient has sarcoidosis. The right radiograph shows the radiological features of fibrosis marked in purple.

Example 3

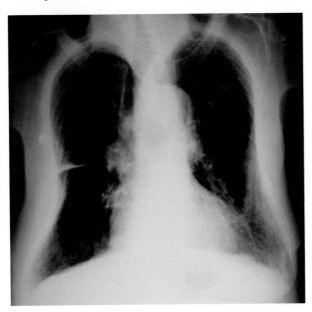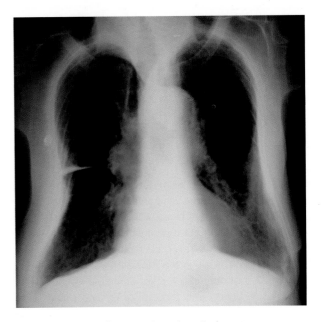

Figure 68 Two identical chest radiographs showing coarse mid- and lower zone fibrosis. There is reticular-type shadowing. The cause is unknown in this radiograph and would have to be determined by the patient's clinical history. The right radiograph shows the radiological features of fibrosis marked in purple. (You can also see: ECG sticker over left upper zone and right chest wall.)

Examples 4, 5, 6 & 7

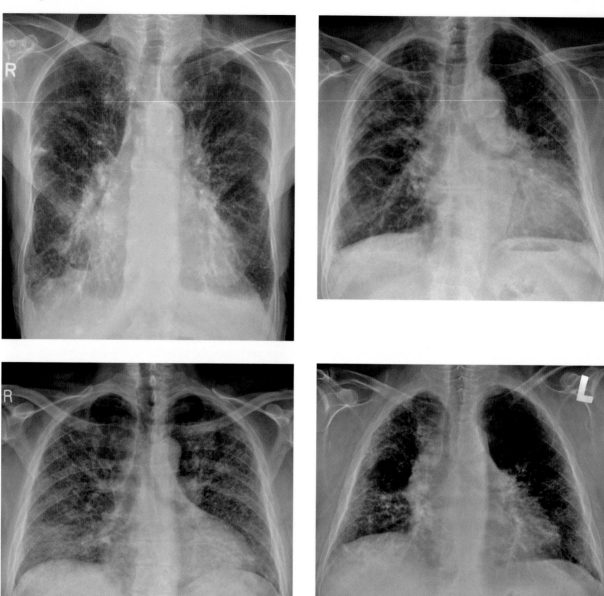

Figure 69 (top left) A chest radiograph showing reticulonodular-type shadowing (fibrosis) throughout both lungs. The cause is unknown in this radiograph and would have to be determined by the patient's clinical history.

Figure 70 (top right) A chest radiograph showing reticulonodular-type shadowing (fibrosis) throughout both lungs. The cause is unknown in this radiograph and would have to be determined by the patient's clinical history.

Figure 71 (bottom left) A chest radiograph showing reticulonodular-type shadowing (fibrosis) throughout both lungs. The cause is unknown in this radiograph and would have to be determined by the patient's clinical history.

Figure 72 (bottom right) A chest radiograph showing reticulonodular-type shadowing (fibrosis) throughout both lungs. The cause is unknown in this radiograph and would have to be determined by the patient's clinical history.

Pneumothorax

A pneumothorax is **air** (seen as black) **in the pleural space**.
1. Parietal pleura
2. Pleural space
3. Visceral pleura
4. Pneumothorax
5. Collapsed lung

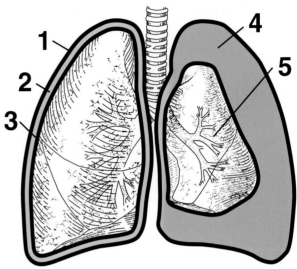

Figure 73 Diagrammatic representation of a left-sided pneumothorax. The air in the pleural space is shown in blue and the normal pleural space is shown in green. In a normal 70 kg man the pleural space contains only a few millilitres of pleural fluid.

A pneumothorax is usually easily seen on a PA chest radiograph. A small pneumothorax may be easier to see on an expiratory film as the reduced volume of the lungs in expiration makes the pneumothorax look relatively larger. The important radiological feature to look for is the **lung edge outlined by air in the pleural space**.

Radiological features to look for
- One side is **blacker** (no lung in it).
  Air in the pleural space causes the lung to recoil to a resting state as the negative pressure in the pleura is lost. The gap left between the lung edge and the parietal pleura is filled with air and appears black on a chest X-ray.
- The **lung edge** is seen and there are **no lung markings beyond the lung edge**.
- Check for **mediastinal shift**.
  Shift of the mediastinum away from the side of the pneumothorax indicates a tension pneumothorax (see p. 56).
- More **prominent vascular markings in the opposite lung**.
  As a pneumothorax causes the affected lung to collapse, most of the right ventricular output is delivered to the opposite lung, leading to increased vascular markings on an erect chest X-ray.

B

Example 1

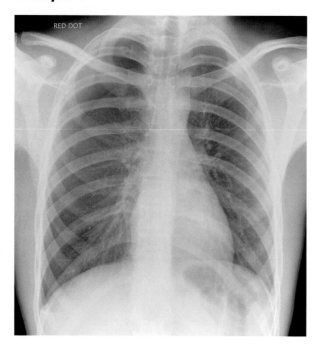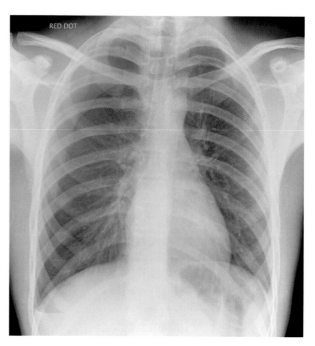

Figure 74 Two identical chest radiographs showing a right pneumothorax. The lung edge is seen and there are no lung markings beyond the lung edge. The vascular markings are more prominent in the opposite lung. The right radiograph shows the pneumothorax marked in blue.

Example 2

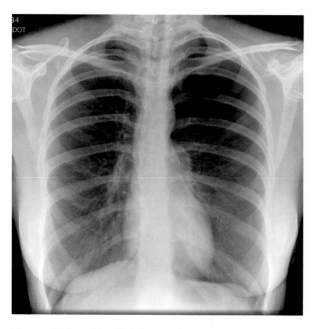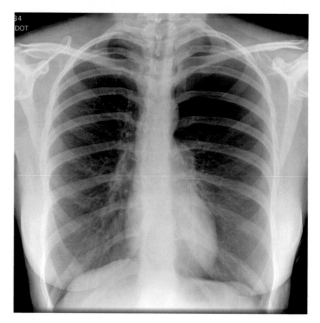

Figure 75 Two identical chest radiographs showing a left pneumothorax. The lung edge is seen and there are no lung markings beyond the lung edge. The vascular markings are more prominent in the opposite lung. The right radiograph shows the pneumothorax marked in blue.

Example 3

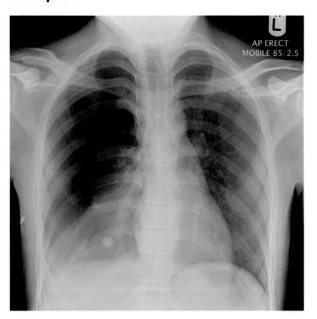
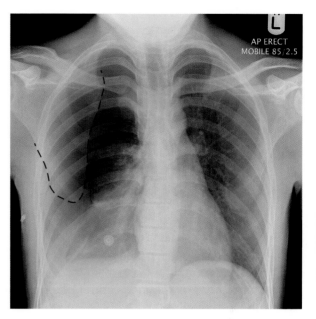

Figure 76 Two identical chest radiographs showing a large right pneumothorax. The lung edge is seen and there are no lung markings beyond the lung edge. The vascular markings are more prominent in the opposite lung. The right radiograph shows the pneumothorax marked in blue. The right scapula is also outlined with a black dotted line to avoid confusion. (You can also see: ECG sticker superimposed on the right lower zone.)

Example 4

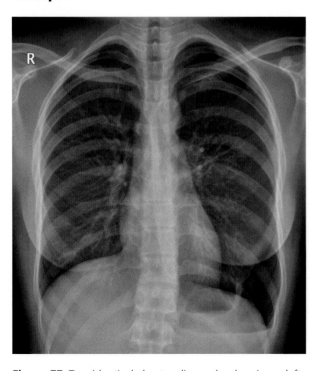
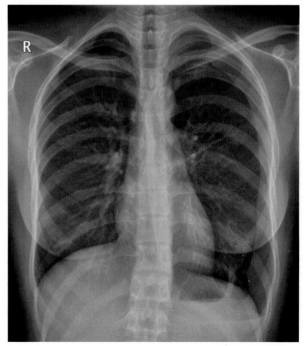

Figure 77 Two identical chest radiographs showing a left pneumothorax. The lung edge is seen and there are no lung markings beyond the lung edge. The vascular markings are more prominent in the opposite lung. The right radiograph shows the pneumothorax marked in blue.

Tension pneumothorax

A tension pneumothorax is a serious type of pneumothorax whereby **air enters but cannot leave** the **pleural space**. This can lead to a complete collapse of the lung and is a medical emergency. It is a **clinical diagnosis**, i.e. it should be diagnosed on history and examination, not radiologically.

Any condition that causes a pneumothorax has the potential to cause a tension pneumothorax. In an uncomplicated pneumothorax, a small amount of air leaks into the pleural space with loss of the normal negative pressure and thus the lung collapses. In a tension pneumothorax, however, air enters the pleural space with each breath causing positive pressure build-up. As the amount of trapped air increases, pressure builds up in the chest and causes the lung to collapse.

Important structures in the centre of the chest (such as the heart, major blood vessels and airways) may be pushed to the other side of the chest. The shift can cause the other lung to become compressed and restrict the pulmonary venous return to the heart resulting in hypoxia, hypotension, shock and rapid death.

Radiological features to look for
- **Darkening** of the hemithorax and **loss of lung markings** due to air in the pleural space.
- **Increased volume** of the hemithorax.
- **Displacement of the mediastinum (and trachea) away** from the pneumothorax.
- **Depressed diaphragm**.

Note: A tension pneumothorax should be diagnosed clinically with shortness of breath, shift of the trachea away from the side of the pneumothorax, hyper-resonance on percussion and reduced or absent breath sounds on auscultation, *not* from a chest radiograph. A delay in treatment could lead to death.

Example 1

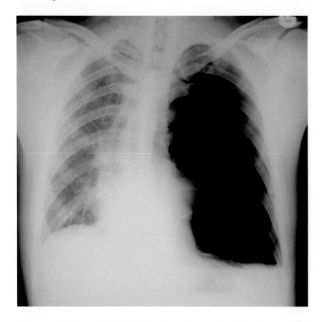 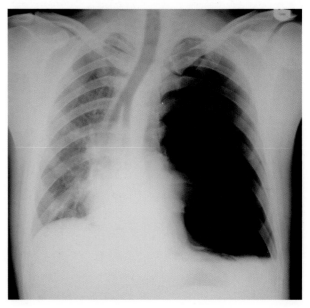

Figure 78 Two identical chest radiographs showing a left tension pneumothorax. There is a depressed left hemidiaphragm, mediastinal shift, right tracheal deviation and loss of normal lung markings as the tension pneumothorax occupies the whole hemithorax. The right radiograph shows the pneumothorax marked in blue.

Example 2

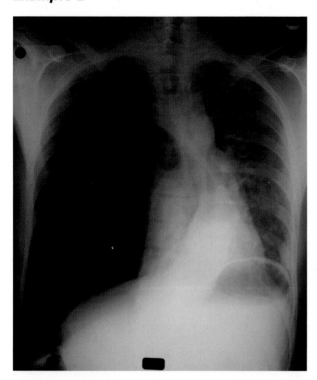
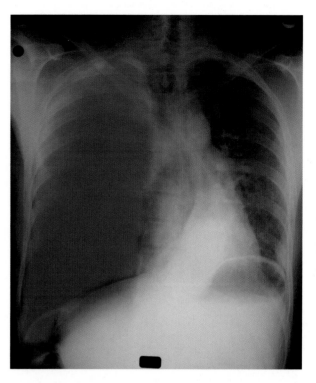

Figure 79 Two identical chest radiographs showing a right tension pneumothorax. The right radiograph shows the pneumothorax marked in blue. There is a depressed right hemidiaphragm and mediastinal shift to the left as the tension pneumothorax occupies the whole hemithorax. There are no lung markings in the space occupied by the tension pneumothorax.

Example 3

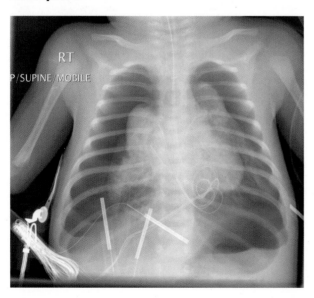
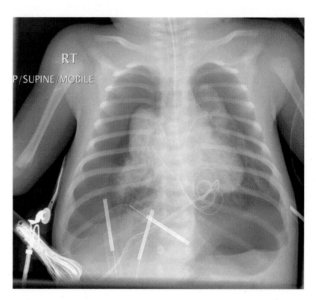

Figure 80 Two identical chest radiographs showing bilateral tension pneumothoraces. The right radiograph shows the pneumothoraces marked in blue. The hemidiaphragms are depressed bilaterally and there are no lung markings in the space occupied by the pneumothorax. Interestingly, there is neither mediastinal shift nor tracheal deviation because there is equal pressure on both sides of the chest, compressing the mediastinum in the middle. The lungs appear denser as they have been compressed to a smaller volume. (You can also see: Endotracheal tube in situ and external cardiac pacing wires.)

> **Note:** A tension pneumothorax is a **'pass or fail'** observation. Always look for this and say, for example:
> 'There is no shift of the mediastinum and therefore tension pneumothorax is unlikely'
> **or**
> 'There is shift of the mediastinum away from the side of the pneumothorax indicating a (right/left) tension pneumothorax. This is a medical emergency, which I would treat immediately by inserting a large bore cannula into the (right/left) pleural space.'

Hydropneumothorax

A **hydropneumothorax** is air and fluid in the pleural space. An erect CXR will show an **air–fluid level**. The horizontal fluid level is usually well defined and extends across the whole length of the hemithorax.

Causes of a hydropneumothorax

- **Iatrogenic**: introduction of air into the pleural space during a pleural fluid aspiration/chest drain insertion in a patient with a pleural effusion.
- **Trauma**.
- **Presence of a gas-forming organism** (rare).

Example 1

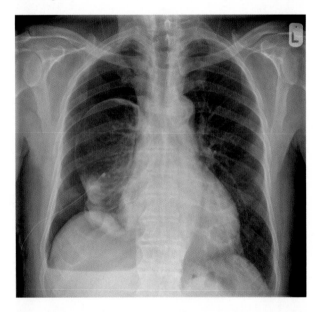 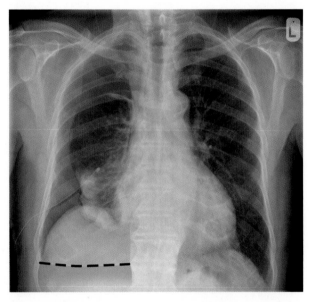

Figure 81 Two identical chest radiographs showing a right-sided hydropneumothorax. The right radiograph shows the pneumothorax marked in blue and the pleural fluid marked in green. The air–fluid level is shown with a black dotted line.

Example 2

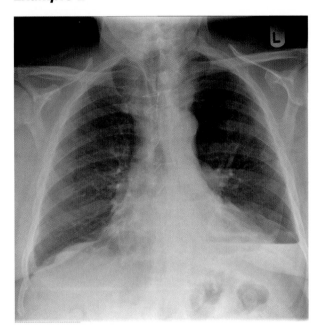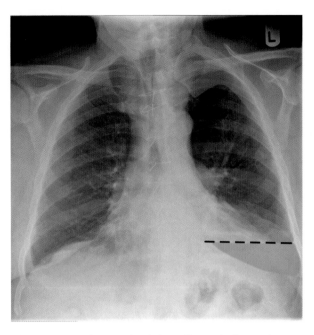

Figure 82 Two identical chest radiographs showing a left-sided hydropneumothorax. The right radiograph shows the pneumothorax marked in blue and the pleural fluid marked in green. The air–fluid level is shown with a black dotted line.

Pleural effusion

A pleural effusion is the **accumulation of fluid** in the **pleural cavity**(the space between the parietal and visceral layers of the pleura).

1. Parietal pleura
2. Pleural space
3. Visceral pleura
4. Pleural effusion

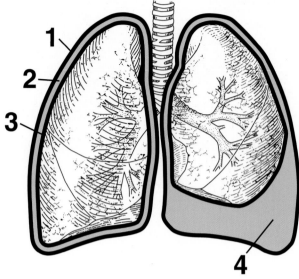

Figure 83 Diagrammatic representation of a left-sided pleural effusion. The pleural space is shown in green. In a normal 70 kg man the intrapleural space contains only a few millilitres of pleural fluid.

This may be caused by the following.

- **Transudate** (<30 g/l of protein):
    - heart failure (congestive heart failure, pericardial effusion)
    - liver failure (cirrhosis)
    - renal failure
    - protein loss (nephrotic syndrome)
    - reduced protein intake (malnutrition)
    - iatrogenic (peritoneal dialysis).
- **Exudate** (>30 g/l of protein):
    - infection (pneumonia, TB)
    - infarction (pulmonary emboli)
    - malignancy (bronchogenic carcinoma, mesothelioma, metastasis)
    - collagen vascular disease (rheumatoid arthritis, systemic lupus erythematosus)
    - pancreatitis (usually left-sided effusion)
    - trauma/surgery (associated with rib fractures).

The X-ray appearances do not change with the nature of the fluid, therefore transudate, exudate, blood (haemothorax), pus or lymph (chylothorax) all look the same. Fluid appears white and on an erect chest X-ray the patient is upright so the fluid from a pleural effusion drains to the bottom of the chest.

> **Note:** Collapse may also cause whiteness at the base of a lung. To help differentiate between collapse and a pleural effusion look at the trachea. With collapse, there is a loss of lung volume and the trachea is deviated towards the affected side. With an effusion, the trachea is usually central (or if massive, may be pushed towards the opposite side). If you suspect pleural effusion, look at the X-ray for a possible cause.

Classical radiological appearance of a pleural effusion
- Homogenous dense opacity (homogenous whiteness).
- Loss of the costophrenic angle.
- Meniscus (i.e. higher laterally than medially), therefore the upper border will be concave.
- Loss of hemidiaphragm.
- No air bronchogram.

Example 1

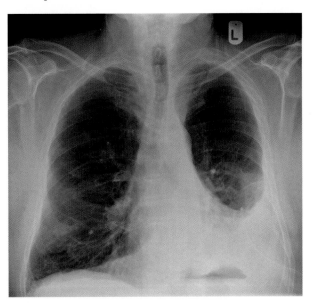 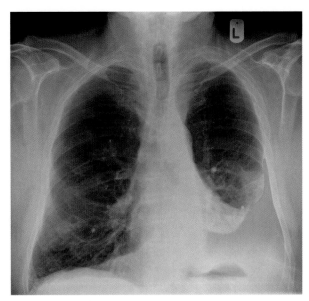

Figure 84 Two identical chest radiographs of a patient with a left-sided pleural effusion. There is a loss of the left costophrenic angle and left hemidiaphragm. The upper edge is concave in shape and a meniscus is seen laterally. The right radiograph shows the pleural effusion marked in green.

Example 2

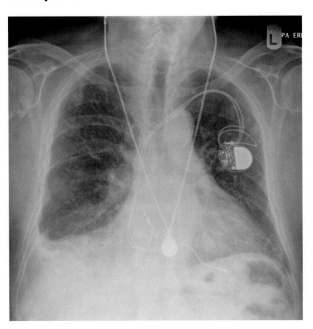 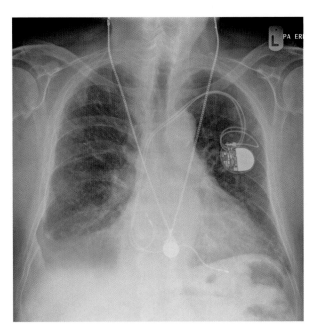

Figure 85 Two identical chest radiographs of a patient with a right-sided pleural effusion. There is a loss of the right costophrenic angle and right hemidiaphragm. The upper edge is concave in shape and a meniscus is seen laterally. The right radiograph shows the pleural effusion marked in green. (You can also see: Cardiac pacemaker with pacing wires in situ and a metal necklace.)

Example 3

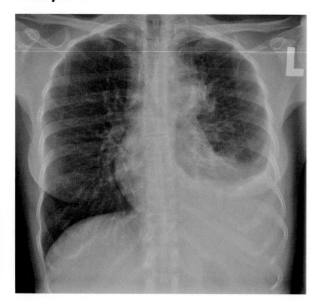 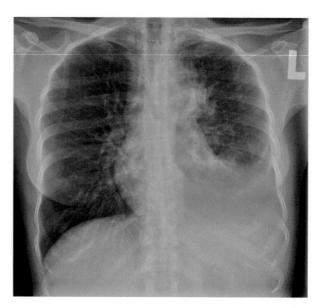

Figure 86 Two identical chest radiographs of a patient with a large left-sided pleural effusion. There is a loss of the left costophrenic angle and left hemidiaphragm. The upper edge is concave in shape and a meniscus is seen laterally. The effusion is a homogenous, dense opacity and there is no air bronchogram. The right radiograph shows the pleural effusion marked in green. The main level of the pleural effusion is marked in dark green; however, it has also tracked up the posterior edge of the lung and up the oblique fissure, creating another level, marked in light green.

Example 4

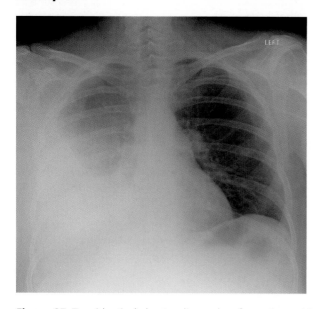 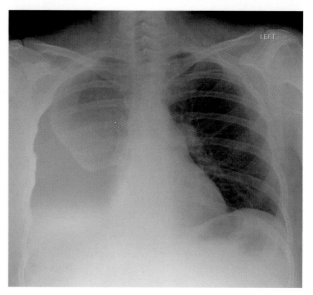

Figure 87 Two identical chest radiographs of a patient with a large right-sided pleural effusion. There is a loss of the right costophrenic angle and right hemidiaphragm. The upper edge is concave in shape and a meniscus is seen laterally. The effusion is a homogenous, dense opacity and there is no air bronchogram. The right radiograph shows the pleural effusion marked in green. The main level of the pleural effusion is marked in dark green; however, it has also tracked up the posterior edge of the lung, creating another level, marked in light green.

Example 5

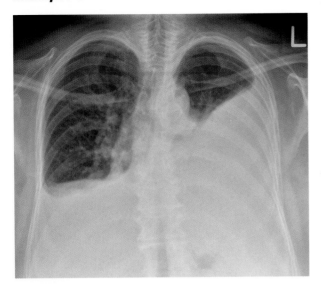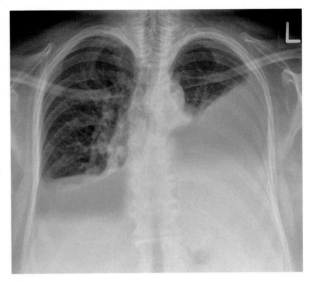

Figure 88 Two identical chest radiographs of a patient with bilateral pleural effusions. The left-sided effusion is larger than the right. There is a loss of the left and right costophrenic angles and hemidiaphragms. The upper edge is concave in shape and a meniscus is seen laterally. The effusion is a homogenous, dense opacity and there is no air bronchogram. The right radiograph shows the pleural effusions marked in green. The main level of the right pleural effusion is marked in dark green; however, it has also tracked up the posterior edge of the lung, creating another level, marked in light green.

Example 6

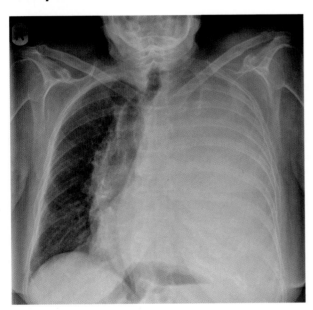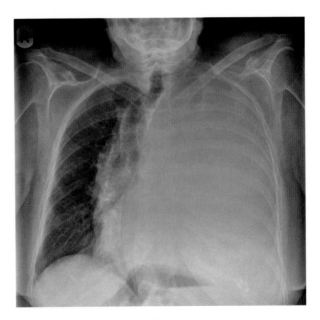

Figure 89 Two identical chest radiographs of a patient with a massive left-sided pleural effusion. There is a loss of the left costophrenic angle and left hemidiaphragm. There is no meniscus as the pleural effusion extends all the way to the apex of the left lung. The effusion is a homogenous, dense opacity and there is no air bronchogram. You can tell that this is a pleural effusion and not lung collapse or a pneumonectomy because there is mass effect, i.e. the trachea and mediastinum are pushed away from the increased density. The right radiograph shows the pleural effusion marked in green.

> **Note:** Massive pleural effusions such as the one in the example above are frequently associated with an underlying mass lesion.

B

Example 7

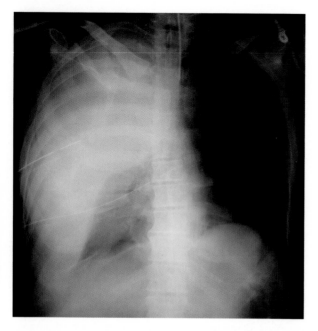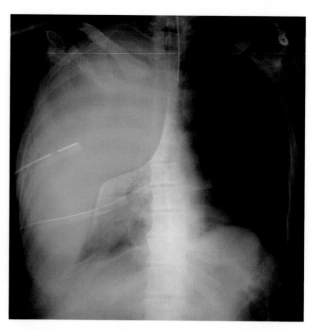

Figure 90 Two identical chest radiographs showing a massive right-sided pleural effusion. There is a loss of the right costophrenic angle and right hemidiaphragm. There is no meniscus as the pleural effusion extends all the way to the apex of the right lung. The effusion is a homogenous, dense opacity and there is no air bronchogram. You can tell that this is a pleural effusion and not lung collapse or a pneumonectomy because there is mass effect, i.e. the trachea and mediastinum are pushed away from the increased density. This patient in fact has a massive haemothorax. There are two chest drains in the right lung to drain the haemothorax. The right radiograph shows the pleural effusion (haemothorax) marked in green. (You can also see: Endotracheal tube in situ and two chest drains.)

Notes on haemothorax

Note: A haemothorax looks the same as a pleural effusion on a chest X-ray.

The cause of a haemothorax is usually traumatic: a blunt or penetrating injury to the thorax results in **rupture of the parietal or visceral pleura**. This rupture allows blood to spill into the pleural space, equalising the pressures between the pleural space and the lungs.

Blood loss into this space may be massive as each hemithorax can hold **30–40%** of a person's blood volume.

Other than trauma, a haemothorax may occur as a complication of:
- **pneumothorax**
- **pulmonary infarct**
- **anticoagulant therapy**, which may potentiate the ability of a chest injury to cause a haemothorax.

Pulmonary oedema

Pulmonary oedema is **fluid accumulation in the lungs** that causes flooding of the alveoli with fluid. This causes severe **disturbance of gas exchange** across the alveolar surface and can lead to respiratory failure.

> **Note:** Pulmonary oedema differs from a pleural effusion because in pulmonary oedema the fluid is in the alveoli and in a pleural effusion the fluid is in the pleural space.

Causes of pulmonary oedema

1. **Cardiogenic pulmonary oedema**
   - **Heart failure**. Failure of the heart to remove fluid from the pulmonary circulation (left ventricular dysfunction or mitral valve disease).
2. **Non-cardiogenic pulmonary oedema**
   - **Renal failure** with fluid overload.
   - **Iatrogenic** fluid overload.
   - **Adult respiratory distress syndrome (ARDS)**.

Radiological appearances

- **Symmetrical, diffuse 'fuzzy' shadowing** (with sparing of the peripheries): especially in the mid- and lower zones where the pulmonary venous pressure is highest due to gravity (provided the patient has been upright).
- **Upper lobe blood diversion**: vessels in upper lobe larger than vessels in lower lobe on erect chest X-ray (due to increased pulmonary vascular resistance in the lower zones).
- **Peribronchial shadowing**: the bronchi are thickened when viewed end-on. This is a radiographic sign occurring when excess fluid builds up in the small airways causing localised patches of atelectasis (lung collapse). This causes the area around the bronchus to appear more prominent on an X-ray.
- **Peri-hilar haziness**: hazy shadowing around the hilar regions.
- In acute cases you may see the characteristic **'bat's wing' pattern** (*see* p. 67).
- **Septal lines** (*see* p. 69).

Example 1

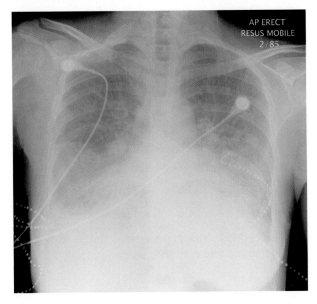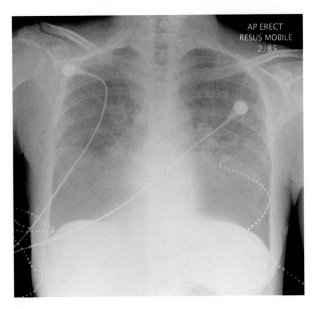

Figure 91 Two identical chest radiographs showing bilateral pulmonary oedema. The right radiograph shows the symmetrical, diffuse 'fuzzy' shadowing of pulmonary oedema marked in pink. (You can also see: Bilateral pleural effusions, ECG leads and the dotted lines are clothing artefacts.)

Example 2

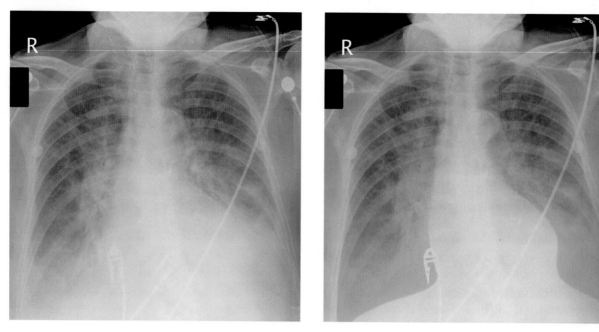

Figure 92 Two identical chest radiographs showing bilateral pulmonary oedema. There is symmetrical, diffuse 'fuzzy' shadowing, particularly in the mid- and lower zones and peri-hilar haziness. The right radiograph shows the pulmonary oedema marked in pink. (You can also see: Bilateral pleural effusions and ECG leads.)

Example 3

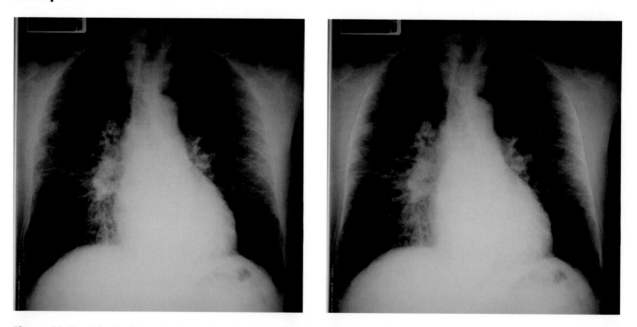

Figure 93 Two identical chest radiographs showing bilateral pulmonary oedema. There is peri-hilar haziness and septal lines. The right radiograph shows peri-hilar haziness marked in pink and septal lines marked in yellow.

'Bat's wing' pattern shadowing

In acute **pulmonary oedema** you may see the radiological appearance of bilateral or unilateral **ill-defined opacities** confined to the **central (peri-hilar) area** of the lungs, **extending laterally to stop 2–3 cm before the periphery of the lung**.

- The opacity takes the shape of a bat's wing (you may have to use your imagination here).
- To date there is no explanation for this distribution of disease, which occurs almost exclusively in patients with **pulmonary oedema**.
- Classically associated with **left ventricular failure** and resultant pulmonary oedema.

Example 1

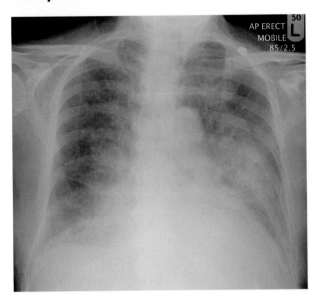 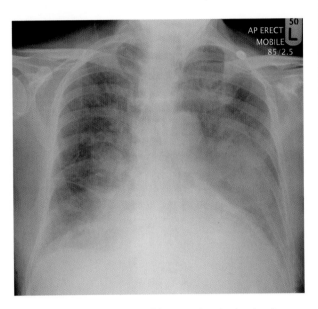

Figure 94 Two identical chest radiographs showing 'bat's wing' pattern of shadowing. In this case the shadowing is unilateral (only on the left side). There is an ill-defined opacity on the left, extending laterally to stop 2–3 cm before the periphery of the lung. The right radiograph shows the 'bat's wing' pattern of shadowing marked in pink. (You can also see: Middle lobe consolidation and other features of pulmonary oedema such as lower zone symmetrical diffuse fuzzy shadowing.)

B

Example 2

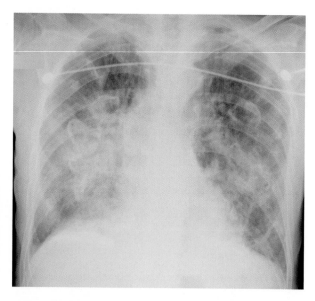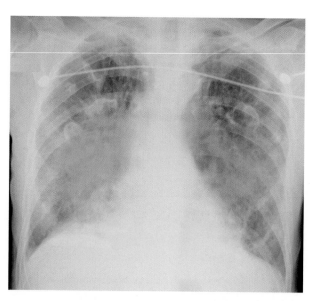

Figure 95 Two identical chest radiographs showing 'bat's wing' pattern of shadowing. In this case the shadowing is bilateral. There are ill-defined opacities extending laterally from the hilar regions of both lungs to stop 3–4 cm before the periphery of the lung. The right radiograph shows the 'bat's wing' pattern of shadowing marked in pink. (You can also see: Calcified pleural plaques throughout both lung fields.)

Septal lines

Septal lines are caused by **engorgement** of the **pulmonary interlobular septal lymphatics** by fluid, tumour or fibrosis.

Septal lines are found around the **periphery** of the lungs, **extending inwards from the pleural surface**. They are invisible on the normal chest radiograph.

They become visible when **thickened** by **fluid, tumour** or **fibrosis**.

On a chest radiograph, the lines are **very fine** and seen around the **peripheries** at a **90° angle** to the pleura. They are easy to miss so *actively* look for them.

> **Note:** Originally described by Kerley, septal lines are traditionally known as **Kerley 'A' lines** (in the central portion of the lung) or **Kerley 'B' lines** (in the periphery of the lung).
> **They should now be collectively referred to as 'septal lines'**.

B

Causes of septal lines

- **Interstitial pulmonary oedema** (e.g. from pulmonary venous hypertension secondary to heart failure).
- **Lymphangitis carcinomatosa**. In advanced malignancy the septal lymphatics may become obstructed or infiltrated by tumour leading to the appearance of septal lines. They are usually bilateral and may be associated with hilar node enlargement.
- **Fibrosis in pneumoconiosis** (very rarely).

Example

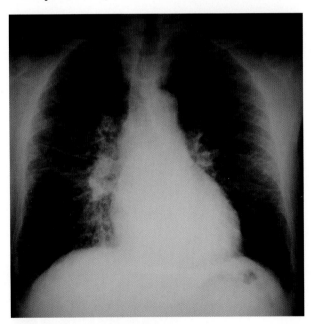 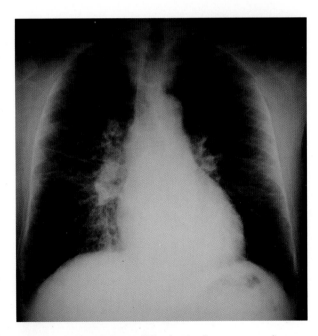

Figure 96a Two identical chest radiographs showing septal lines (associated with heart failure). The lines are very fine and are seen around the peripheries at a 90° angle to the chest wall. The right radiograph highlights the septal lines in yellow.

B

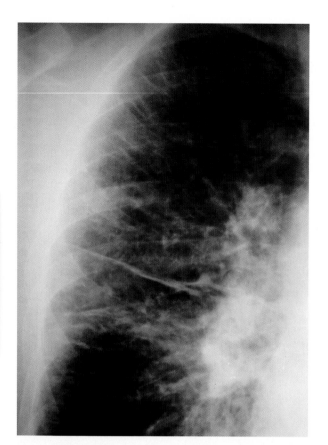
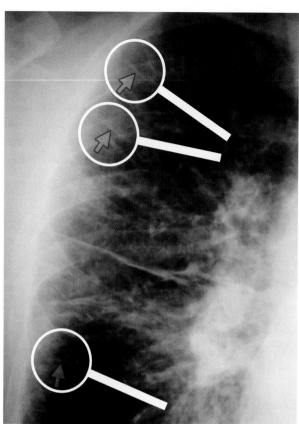

Figure 96b Two identical chest radiographs (the same radiograph as Figure 96a) showing many septal lines in the right lung. The lines are very fine and are seen in the peripheries at a 90° angle to the chest wall. The right radiograph shows three of the septal lines marked with yellow arrows.

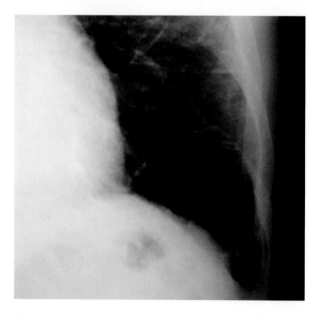
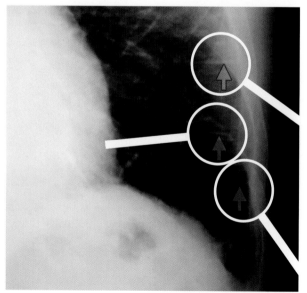

Figure 96c Two identical chest radiographs (the same radiograph as Figure 96a) showing many septal lines in the left lower zone. The lines are very fine and are seen in the peripheries at a 90° angle to the chest wall. The right radiograph shows three of the septal lines marked with yellow arrows.

Dextrocardia

Dextrocardia literally means that the heart is arranged in a **perfect mirror image** to the normal positioning. Therefore the heart is in the **right hemithorax**, with the **cardiac apex directed to the right**. Basically the heart is the wrong way round.

In some patients, all the visceral organs of the chest are mirrored (heart and lungs, etc.) and are arranged in the exact opposite position. This is called dextrocardia situs inversus totalis. In dextrocardia situs inversus totalis the heart and two-lobed lung are both on the right and the three-lobed lung is on the left. As this arrangement is a perfect mirror image, the relationship between the organs is not changed.

> **Note:** ECG leads and defibrillation pads must be placed in reversed positions on a person with dextrocardia.

Example

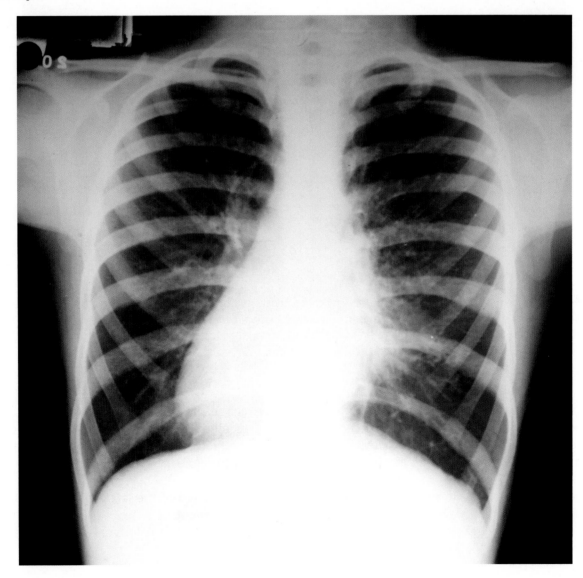

Figure 97 An erect chest radiograph showing dextrocardia. The heart is in the right hemithorax with its apex directed to the right.

Cardiomegaly (enlarged heart)

If the width of the heart is **more than half the total width of the thorax**, the patient has cardiomegaly. The width should be measured horizontally and is the longest possible distance between the left and right heart borders.

> **Note:** You can *only* comment on the cardiac size on a PA (posterior–anterior) chest radiograph. This is because on AP (antero–posterior) or *supine* radiographs the mediastinum and cardiac size will appear wider due to venous distension and magnification (*see* p. 4). Therefore you *should not* comment on the cardiac or mediastinal size on an AP/supine film.

Example

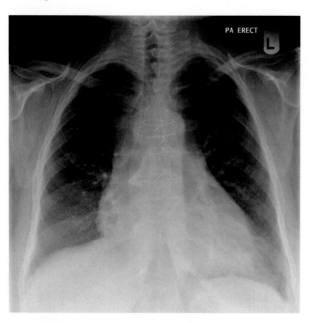 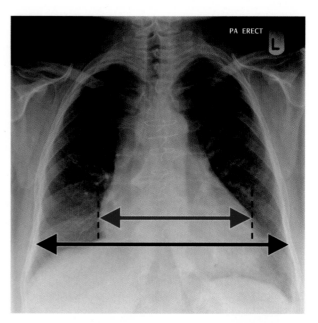

Figure 98 Two identical PA chest radiographs showing cardiomegaly. The black dotted lines mark the edge of the heart. The shorter red arrow marks the width of the heart. The longer black arrow marks the width of the thoracic cavity. The width of the heart is greater than half the width of the thoracic cavity, therefore the heart is enlarged (cardiomegaly). (You can also see: Median sternotomy wires.)

Normally two-thirds of the heart should lie to the left of the midline and one-third to the right of the midline. The left ventricle forms the left heart border and the right atrium forms the right heart border. Both the left atrium and right ventricle are not visible on the normal chest radiograph. This is because the right ventricle lies anteriorly and the left atrium lies posteriorly, and they therefore have no definable border on a chest X-ray.

The image of the heart that you see on the PA CXR is **mainly comprised of the left ventricle**, therefore in cardiomegaly, what you are actually seeing is **left ventricle enlargement**.

The most common reason for the heart to be enlarged is **heart failure**, so look for signs of left ventricular failure on the rest of the film (*see* Heart failure, p. 95).

Left atrial enlargement

The left atrium may be seen on a PA chest X-ray as the **left atrial appendage**. The left atrial appendage is normally concave in shape, but if the left atrium is enlarged (usually secondary to **mitral stenosis**) there is a **loss of concavity and straightening of the left atrial appendage**. Sometimes atrial enlargement is so great that the left atrial appendage bulges outwards.

Radiological signs due to left atrial enlargement
- **Straightening or bulging** of the **left atrial appendage**.
- **Widening** of the **carinal angle** (*see* p. 22).
- May see a **double shadow** at the **right heart border** due to left atrial dilatation.

Example

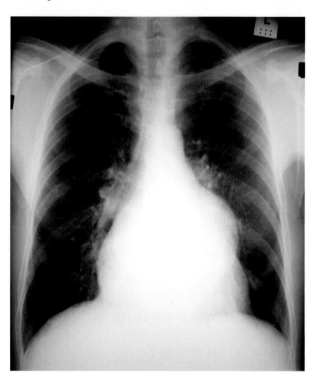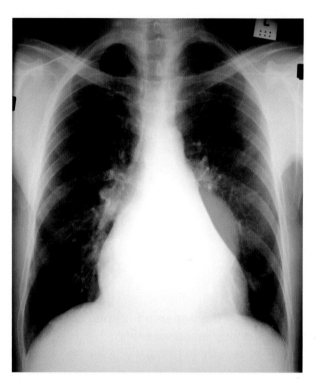

Figure 99 Two identical chest radiographs showing left atrial enlargement. In this case the left atrium is enlarged secondary to mitral valve disease. The left atrial appendage is bulging out and the right heart border appears further over to the right than usual. The right radiograph shows the left atrial appendage marked in red.

Widened mediastinum

The mediastinum is the **central part of the thorax**. It contains the heart, the great vessels, oesophagus, trachea, phrenic nerve, vagus nerve, sympathetic chain, thoracic duct, thymus and central lymph nodes (including hilar lymph nodes). If you think the mediastinum is wider than normal, relate this finding to the patient's clinical history. **Hilar enlargement also gives a widened mediastinum** and is covered in a separate section on pages 77–78.

Note: Always check to ensure the film is not rotated. A rotated film can make the mediastinum look widened.

Important causes of a widened mediastinum:
- aortic dilatation (aortic aneurysm or dissection)
- lymph node enlargement
- dilatation of the oesophagus
- thyroid enlargement
- thymic tumours.

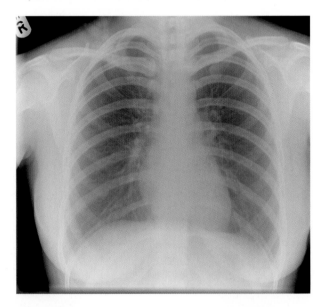

Figure 100 A normal chest radiograph showing the mediastinum marked in orange.

The level of the widening (upper, central, lower) can help determine the cause.
- Upper mediastinal widening:
  - more likely to be paratracheal lymphadenopathy, thyroid or thymus in origin.
- Central or lower mediastinal widening:
  - more likely to be hilar enlargement, aortic widening, lymphadenopathy, dilatation of the oesophagus or a thymic tumour.

Radiological signs to look for
- **If you suspect widening of the aorta:**
  - follow its outline. You may see a continuous edge that widens to form the edge of the enlarged mediastinum
  - look for calcification in the wall of the aorta and if you can see a line of calcium, follow it
    - if the calcified aortic wall bulges, there is likely to be an aortic aneurysm
    - if the line of calcium separates from the edge of the aortic shadow then this would be in keeping with an aortic dissection.

Note: The aorta may become tortuous in the elderly and this may mimic a widened aorta.

- **If you suspect an enlarged thyroid:**
  - look at the position of the trachea. An enlarged thyroid will displace or narrow the trachea.

Example 1

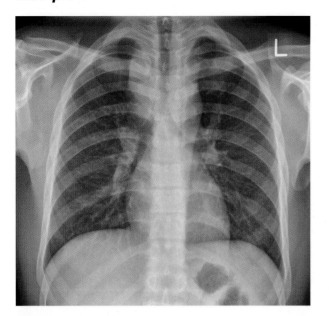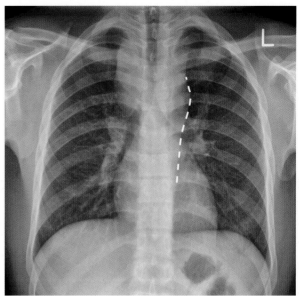

Figure 101 Two identical chest radiographs showing paratracheal lymph node enlargement. The upper mediastinum looks widened with a smooth lobular appearance. The right radiograph shows the paratracheal lymph nodes marked in orange. The outline of the descending thoracic aorta is marked with a white dotted line. Do not confuse the descending thoracic aorta with lymph node enlargement. You can tell it is the aorta as the outline continues inferiorly down the length of the thorax.

Example 2

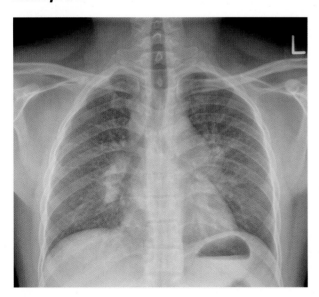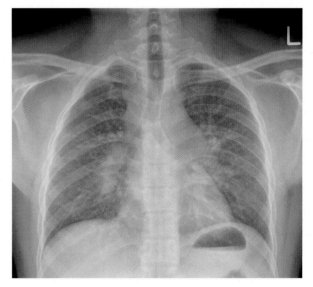

Figure 102 Two identical chest radiographs showing hilar and paratracheal lymph node enlargement. The central and upper mediastinum looks widened with a smooth lobular appearance. The right radiograph shows the paratracheal and hilar lymph nodes marked in orange.

C

Example 3

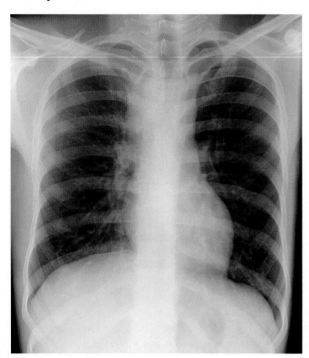 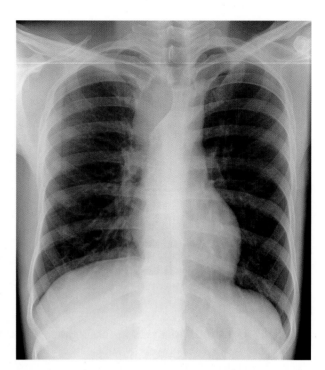

Figure 103 Two identical chest radiographs showing right paratracheal lymph node enlargement. The upper mediastinum looks widened with a smooth lobular appearance. The trachea is actually deviated to the left – being pushed over by the enlarged lymph node. The right radiograph shows the paratracheal lymph node marked in orange. In this case the likely cause of unilateral lymph node enlargement could be TB or a primary lymphoma.

C

Hilar enlargement

Suspect hilar enlargement if:
- one hilum is **bigger** than the other
- one hilum is **denser** than the other
- there is **loss of the normal concave shape** (this may be the first sign of hilar enlargement).

Each hilar complex as seen on a PA chest radiograph consists of the:
1. **Pulmonary artery**
2. **Bronchus**
3. **Lymph nodes** (not visible unless enlarged)
4. **Superior and inferior pulmonary veins**

In assessing hilar enlargement you must decide which of these structures are involved. Hilar enlargement always requires further investigation.

The three causes of unilateral hilar enlargement
1. **Enlarged vascular shadows**
   - If the branching pulmonary arteries are seen to arise from an apparent mass, this would indicate an enlarged main pulmonary artery.
   - Vascular margins are usually smooth in nature.

Causes: Pulmonary artery aneurysm or post-stenotic dilatation of the pulmonary artery.

2. **Enlargement of the hilar lymph nodes (lymphadenopathy)**
   - Smooth lobular appearance.
   - Presence of calcium deposits (very bright white).
   - Look at the periphery for lung lesions (tumour, TB).
   - Look at the rest of the mediastinum. Malignant hilar enlargement may be associated with superior mediastinal lymphadenopathy.

Causes: Infection (e.g. TB), spread from primary lung tumour, primary lymphoma or sarcoidosis (rarely unilateral).

3. **Central bronchial carcinoma superimposed over the hilar shadow**
   - Spiculated, irregular or indistinct margins.
   - Look at the periphery for other lung lesions (tumours) or bony lesions (metastasis).
   - Look at the rest of the mediastinum. Malignant hilar enlargement may be associated with superior mediastinal lymphadenopathy.

C

The two causes of bilateral *hilar enlargement*

1. Pulmonary hypertension

- Pulmonary arterial enlargement is a cause of bilateral hilar enlargement. If the branching pulmonary arteries are seen to arise from an apparent mass, this would indicate an enlarged main pulmonary artery.
- May be associated with reduction in the peripheral vascularity. The edge of the lung fields are often darker than usual and the central area often whiter (this is often associated with congenital heart disease).
- Look for a cause (e.g. signs of mitral stenosis or features of chronic lung disease).

Causes: Obstructive lung disease (e.g. asthma, COPD), left heart disease (e.g. mitral stenosis, LVF), left to right shunts (e.g. ASD, VSD), recurrent pulmonary emboli or primary pulmonary hypertension.

2. Bilateral enlargement of the hilar lymph nodes (lymphadenopathy)

- Smooth lobular appearance.
- Presence of calcium deposits (very bright white).
- Look at the periphery for lung lesions (tumour, TB, fibrosis).
- Look at the rest of the mediastinum. Malignant hilar enlargement may be associated with superior mediastinal lymphadenopathy.

Causes: Sarcoidosis, infection (e.g. TB), spread from primary lung tumour or primary lymphoma.

Hiatus hernia

A hiatus hernia is the **herniation of the stomach into the thorax**. On an erect chest X-ray it appears as a 'mass' behind the heart with an **air–fluid level**.

Example 1

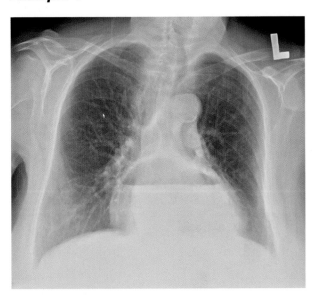 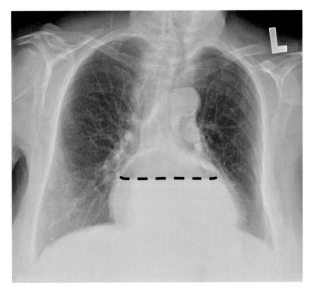

Figure 104 Two identical chest radiographs showing a hiatus hernia. The right radiograph shows the gastric contents in yellow and the gastric air bubble in blue. The air–fluid level is shown with a black dotted line. (You can also see: Widening of the carinal angle due to the size of the hiatus hernia.)

Example 2

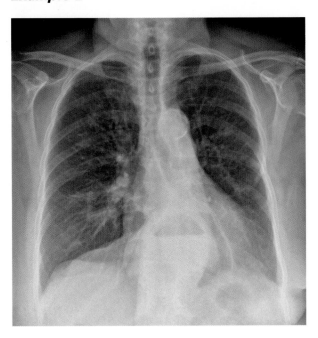 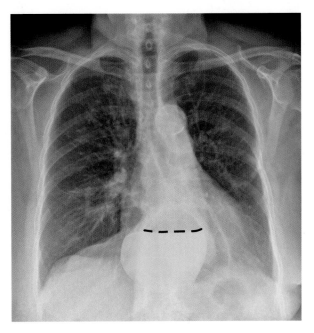

Figure 105 Two identical chest radiographs showing a hiatus hernia. The right radiograph shows the gastric contents in yellow and the gastric air bubble in blue. The air–fluid level is shown with a black dotted line.

C

Rib fractures and other bony abnormalities

Rib fractures are much easier to see if you **rotate the radiograph through 90°**.

> **Note:** This is because when you look at a radiograph normally, your eyes are trained to look at the anatomy of the lungs and heart, etc. However, rotating the image tricks your brain, and your eyes tend to focus on the more dense parts (ribs and other bones), making it easier to spot a fracture or bony abnormality.

- **Step closer** to the radiograph and **follow the edges** of each bone to look for **fractures**. Look for areas of **blackness** and **compare** the density of the bones on **both sides**. They should be the same. Look for destruction, spurs and degenerative changes.
- **Are all the ribs present**? If not, they may have been removed during a previous thoracotomy.
- **Are the vertebrae intact**? Look for compression fractures.

Example 1

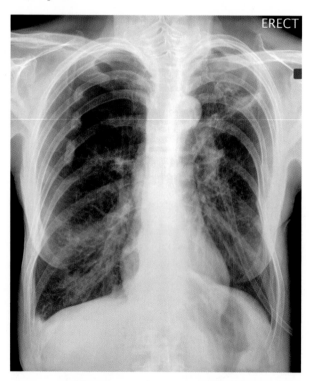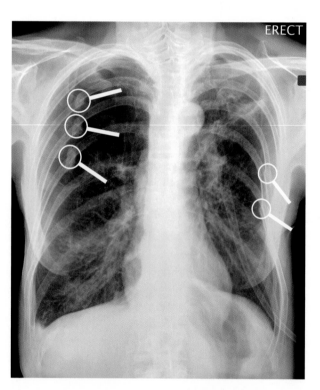

Figure 106 Two identical chest radiographs showing rib fractures. There are five rib fractures seen. The 5th, 6th and 7th right ribs are fractured posteriorly with some callus formation (indicating they are a few weeks old and healing). The 6th and 7th left ribs are also fractured posteriorly. This patient in fact has a flail chest – a potentially life-threatening medical condition. The right radiograph shows all five rib fractures surrounded by white circles. (You can also see: Oxygen mask tubing overlying the left hemithorax.)

Example 2

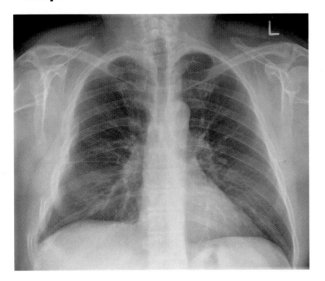
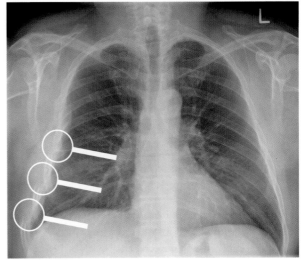

Figure 107 Two identical chest radiographs showing lytic bone metastases. There are lytic areas in each of the 6th, 7th and 8th ribs. The right radiograph shows each area of bone lysis surrounded by a white circle.

Example 3

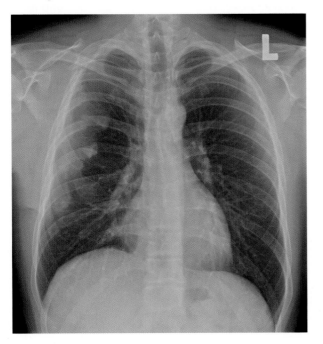
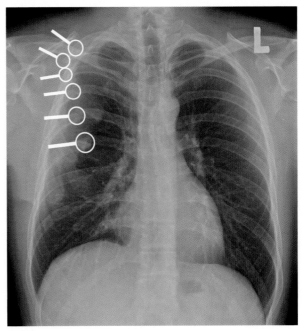

Figure 108 Two identical chest radiographs showing rib fractures. There are six rib fractures seen. The 2nd, 3rd, 4th, 5th, 6th and 7th right ribs are fractured posteriorly. The right radiograph shows all six rib fractures surrounded by white circles.

D

Air under the diaphragm (pneumoperitoneum)

Pneumoperitoneum literally means **free air in the peritoneal cavity**. It indicates **perforation of an intra-abdominal hollow viscus**. It may also be seen soon after laparotomy and laparoscopy.

On an **erect** chest radiograph you will see the **free air under the diaphragm**. It appears as a **rim of blackness** beneath and very **closely opposed** to the curve of the diaphragm. The erect chest X-ray is a **very sensitive** investigation for **detecting free abdominal air** since it can detect as little as **10 ml**.

> **Note:** Normally the area immediately under the diaphragm is white, since the upper part of the abdomen contains the dense structures of the liver and spleen. Because of this you can usually only make out the upper surface of the diaphragm. A pneumoperitoneum may enable you to see both the upper and lower surface of the diaphragm.

> **Note:** A subphrenic abscess (abscess under the diaphragm) may mimic a pneumoperitoneum if there is a gas-forming organism associated with it.

Main causes of intra-abdominal perforation
- Perforated peptic ulcer.
- Perforated appendix/bowel/bowel diverticulum.
- Post-surgery.
- Trauma.

You may see a darker area under the left hemidiaphragm. This is the air bubble within the stomach and is normal. To differentiate between a pneumoperitoneum and the normal stomach bubble look at the following.
- **The thickness of the diaphragm**: if there is air immediately below the diaphragm, the white line of the diaphragm between the air and the chest will be very thin as it will consist of the diaphragm only. If the air is in the stomach, the white line will be thicker as it will consist of the diaphragm and the stomach lining.
- **Length of the air bubble**: the distance from its medial to its lateral aspect. If longer than half the length of the hemidiaphragm, then it is likely to be free air, as air within the stomach is restricted by the anatomy of the stomach.
- **Is there air bilaterally?** If air is present below the left and right hemidiaphragms, it is likely to be free air in the abdomen.

> **Note:** If still in doubt, take another X-ray but with the patient on their side. Free abdominal air will rise away from the diaphragm to the uppermost aspect of the abdomen, whereas air within the stomach will remain in the same place.

E

Example 1

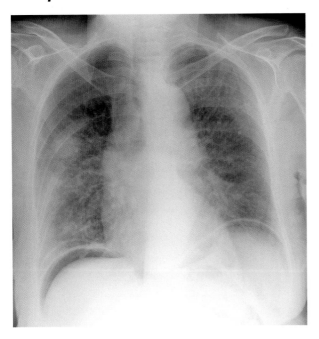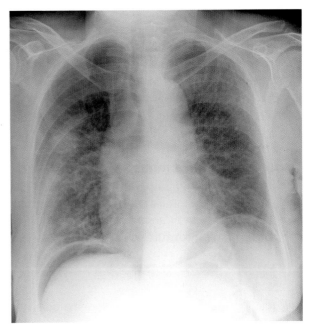

Figure 109 Two identical erect chest radiographs showing air under the diaphragm (pneumoperitoneum). Note that the white line of the diaphragm between the free air in the abdomen and the lungs is very thin. The distance from the medial to lateral aspect of the air bubble is over half the length of the hemidiaphragm, reducing the probability that this appearance is due to air within the stomach or bowel. There is also air bilaterally, increasing the likelihood that this is a pneumoperitoneum. The right radiograph shows the air under the diaphragm marked in blue. (You can also see: Oxygen mask tubing and a mass lesion in the right lung.)

Example 2

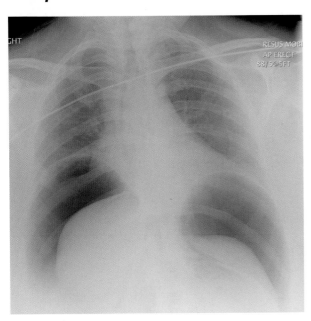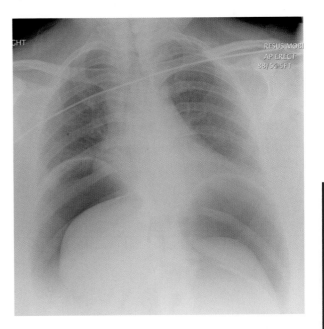

Figure 110 Two identical erect chest radiographs showing air under the diaphragm (pneumoperitoneum). Note that the white line of the diaphragm between the free air in the abdomen and the lungs is very thin. The distance from the medial to lateral aspect of the air bubble is over half the length of the hemidiaphragm, reducing the probability that this appearance is due to air within the stomach or bowel. There is also air bilaterally, increasing the likelihood that this is a pneumoperitoneum. The right radiograph shows the air under the diaphragm marked in blue.

E

Subcutaneous emphysema/surgical emphysema

Emphysema is the abnormal **distension of tissues** caused by the **retention of air**.
- **Subcutaneous emphysema** occurs when air is present in the subcutaneous layer of the skin. On a radiograph there is blackness where there should be whiteness.
- **Surgical emphysema** is the term given when the subcutaneous emphysema is due to surgery.

Subcutaneous/surgical emphysema has a characteristic crackling feel, a sensation that has been described as similar to touching Rice Krispies. This sensation of air under the skin is known as subcutaneous crepitation.

Causes of subcutaneous/surgical emphysema
- **Trauma** (puncture of parts of the respiratory or gastrointestinal systems, particularly in the chest and neck, may result in air becoming trapped under the skin).
- **Pneumothorax** or an **improperly functioning chest drain**.
- **Oesophageal rupture**.

Note: Subcutaneous/surgical emphysema does not usually require any treatment as it resolves spontaneously.

E

Example 1

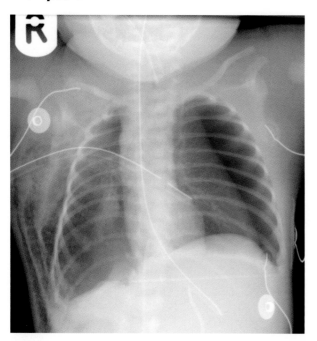 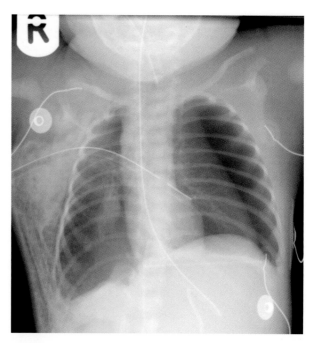

Figure 111 Two identical chest radiographs showing surgical emphysema. The right radiograph shows the surgical emphysema marked in yellow. (You can also see: Left pneumothorax, endotracheal tube in situ, nasogastric tube in situ and ECG leads.)

Example 2

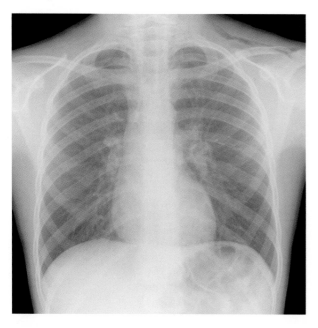 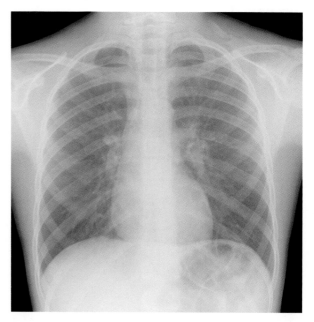

Figure 112 Two identical chest radiographs showing subcutaneous emphysema. In this case the patient was asthmatic and coughed violently, rupturing a bulla or bleb and allowing air from the lung to escape into the mediastinum. The air then tracked upwards to the right shoulder. The right radiograph shows the subcutaneous emphysema marked in yellow.

E

Example 3

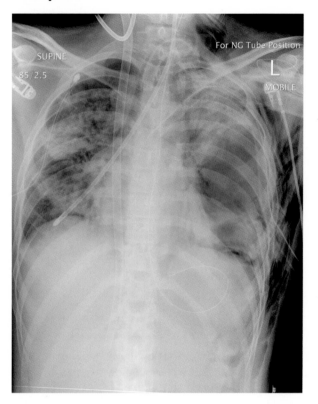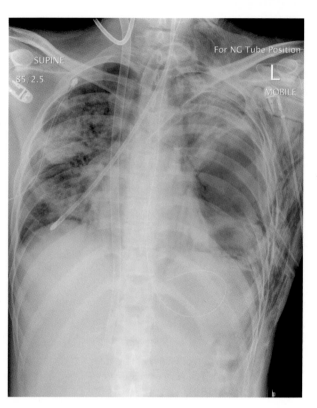

Figure 113 Two identical chest radiographs showing surgical emphysema. The right radiograph shows the surgical emphysema marked in yellow. (You can also see: Bilateral consolidation, tracheostomy tube in situ, ECG leads, extracorporal membrane oxygenation (ECMO) cannula, left pneumothorax and chest drain, and malpositioned nasogastric tube.)

Example 4

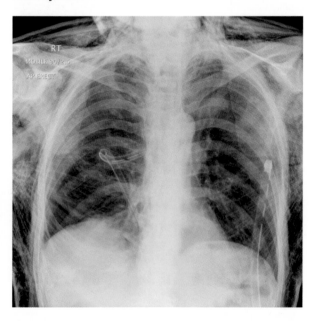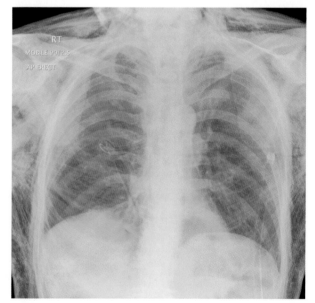

Figure 114 Two identical chest radiographs showing surgical emphysema. The surgical emphysema is extensive and covers most of the thorax. If you look carefully you can see the fibres of pectoralis major. The right radiograph shows the surgical emphysema marked in yellow. (You can also see: Two chest drains in situ.)

Mastectomy

It is important to remember that problems outside the lung can sometimes cause the lung fields to look too black (or too white). A mastectomy is the surgical removal of one or both breasts and will make the **underlying lung look too black** since there will be **less soft tissue overlying** the lung on the affected side, compared to the normal side.

Therefore if one lung looks blacker than the other, look carefully for the breast shadows. There will be an absent breast shadow on the side of the mastectomy.

Example 1

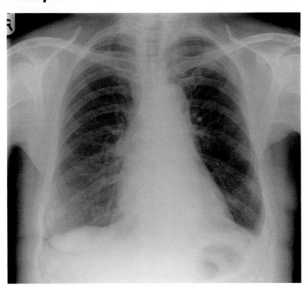 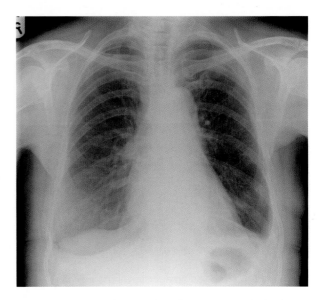

Figure 115 Two identical chest radiographs showing a left mastectomy. The lung field in the left lower zone looks 'blacker' than the lung field in the right lower zone as there is no breast tissue on the left side. The right radiograph shows the right breast marked in pink.

Example 2

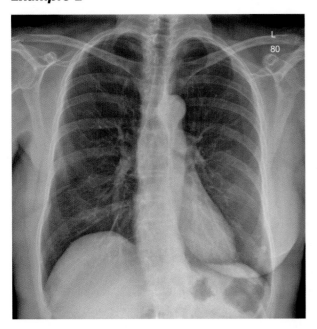 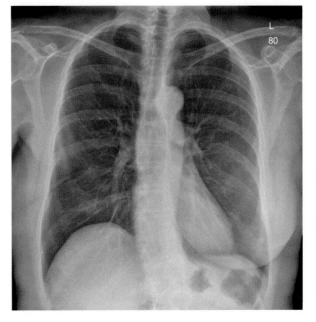

Figure 116 Two identical chest radiographs showing a right mastectomy. The lung field in the right lower zone looks 'blacker' than the lung field in the left lower zone as there is no breast tissue on the right side. The right radiograph shows the left breast marked in pink.

Foreign bodies and medical interventions

There are a number of common examples that you should be able to recognise.

Artificial heart valve

Example 1

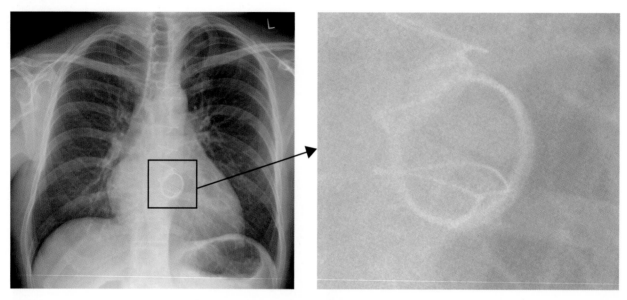

Figure 117 A chest radiograph showing a mechanical heart valve. The valve appears white because it contains metal and therefore absorbs X-rays, leaving a shadow on the film. (You can also see: Median sternotomy wires.)

Example 2

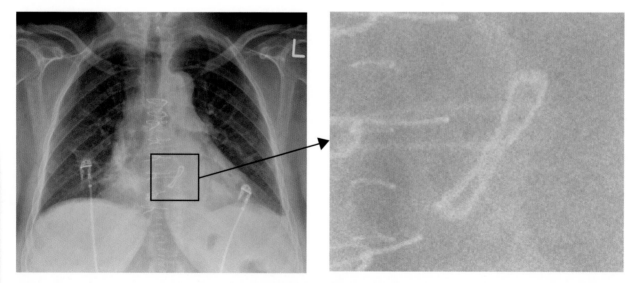

Figure 118 A chest radiograph showing a mechanical heart valve. The valve appears white because it contains metal and therefore absorbs X-rays, leaving a shadow on the film. We know this valve replacement operation was performed recently because we can still see surgical staples (skin closure) running down the midline. (You can also see: Two ECG leads, cardiomegaly, median sternotomy wires and surgical staples.)

E

Breast implants

Example

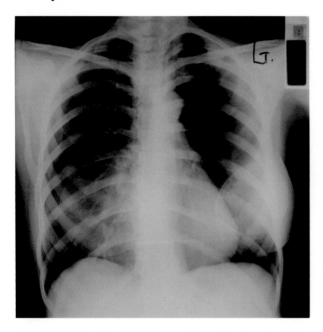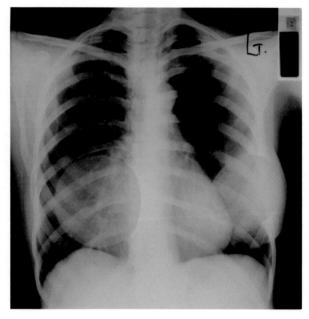

Figure 119 Two identical chest radiographs showing bilateral breast implants. The right radiograph shows the breast implants marked in pink.

Cardiac pacemakers

Example

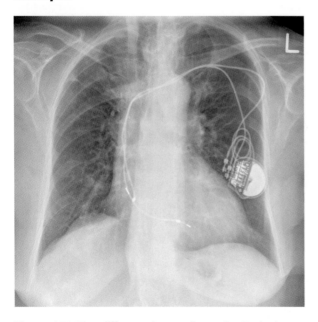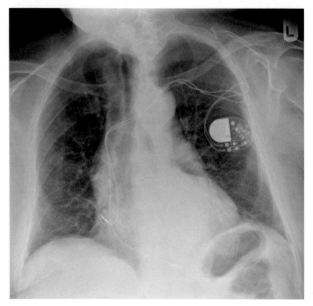

Figure 120 Two different chest radiographs. Both show cardiac pacemakers.

E

Median sternotomy wires (from a previous median sternotomy)

Example

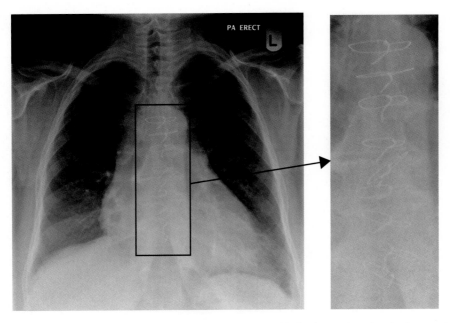

Figure 121 A chest radiograph showing median sternotomy wires. It is likely this patient has had a previous coronary artery bypass craft (CABG). (You can also see: Cardiomegaly.)

Coin stuck in the oesophagus

Example

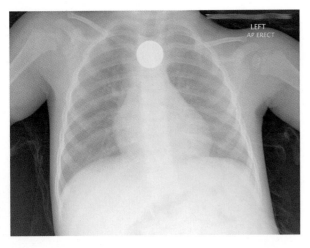 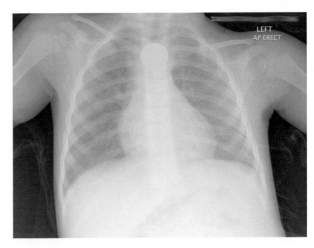

Figure 122 Two identical chest radiographs showing a swallowed coin stuck in the oesophagus of a child. The right radiograph shows the coin marked in yellow.

Nasogastric (NG) tube

Example 1

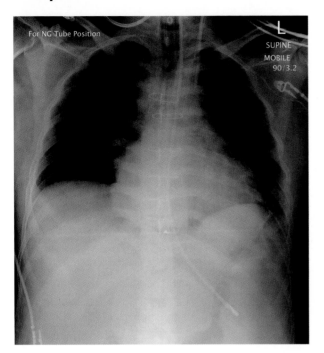 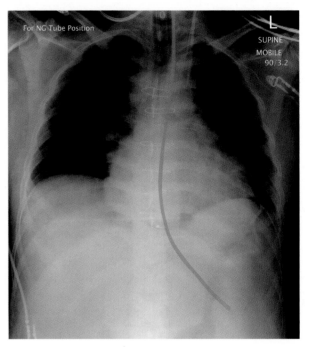

Figure 123 Two identical chest radiographs. The right radiograph shows the NG tube marked in pink. Note that the radiograph was actually taken to assess NG tube position. The NG tube is in the correct position as the tip is clearly beneath the diaphragm. (You can also see: Median sternotomy wires, ECG leads, endotracheal tube in situ and two left internal jugular lines.)

Example 2

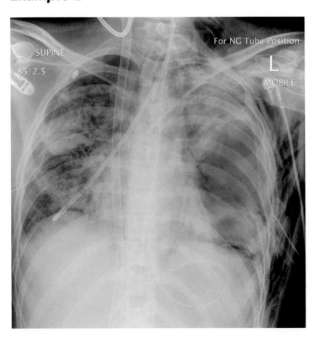 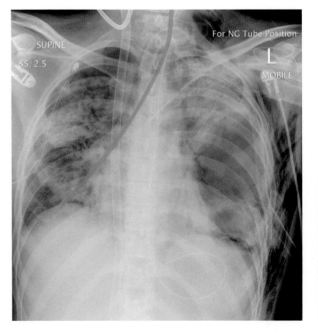

Figure 124 Two identical chest radiographs. The right radiograph shows the NG tube marked in pink. Note that the radiograph was taken to assess NG tube position. The NG tube is malpositioned as it has travelled down the trachea, right mainstem bronchus and intermediate bronchus to end up in the right inferior lobe bronchus. It will need to be repositioned. (You can also see: Bilateral consolidation, subcutaneous emphysema, tracheostomy tube in situ, ECG leads, extracorporal membrane oxygenation (ECMO) cannula, left pneumothorax and chest drain.)

E

Example 3

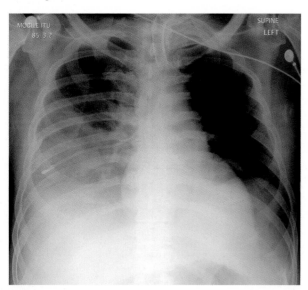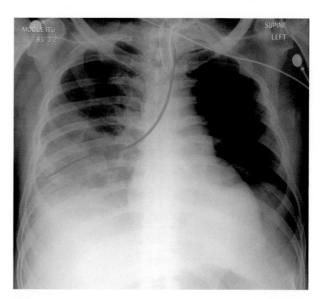

Figure 125 Two identical chest radiographs. The right radiograph shows the NG tube marked in pink. The NG tube is malpositioned as it has travelled down the trachea, right mainstem bronchus and intermediate bronchus to end up in the middle lobe bronchus. It will need to be repositioned. (You can also see: Right lower lobe consolidation, tracheostomy tube in situ and ECG leads.)

E

Tracheostomy tube

Example

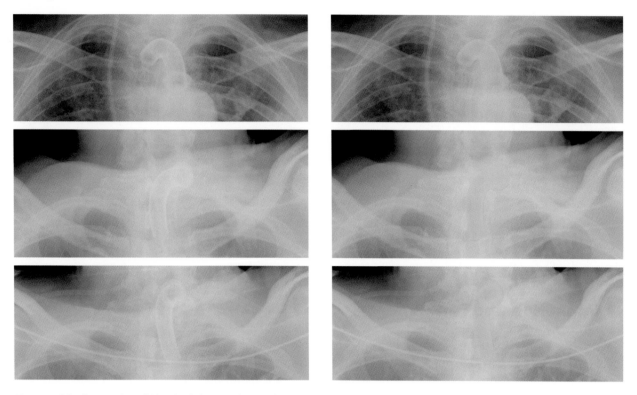

Figure 126 Three pairs of identical chest radiographs, cropped so that only the trachea and apices of the lungs are shown. In each radiograph there is a tracheostomy tube in situ. The right radiographs show the tracheostomy tubes marked in orange.

Loop recorder or Reveal device

Example

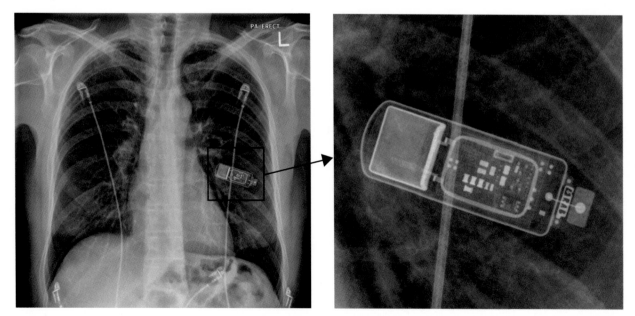

Figure 127 A chest radiograph showing a loop recorder that has been placed subcutaneously on the anterior chest wall. This device may pick up arrhythmias when they occur and is subsequently interrogated by an external reading device.

E

Common conditions and their radiological signs

You must know the following common conditions and their radiological signs.

Pulmonary embolism

> **Note:** There are no specific radiological features of pulmonary embolism on a plain chest X-ray and although some associated features are described (e.g. linear atelectasis and localised oligaemia), they are so inconsistent and ambiguous as to be unhelpful. A plain radiograph may be performed to look for other conditions that mimic pulmonary embolism in their clinical presentation but is not used for its diagnosis.
>
> **The current 'Gold Standard' for the diagnosis of pulmonary embolism is a CT pulmonary angiogram (CTPA)**.

Bronchial carcinoma

This is a common primary tumour, with approximately half found in the peripheral lung fields and half found centrally. The main histological types are: squamous, small cell, anaplastic, adenocarcinoma and alveolar cell carcinoma (rare).

Radiological features
- **Lobulated** or **spiculated mass** but sometimes with a smooth outline.
- May be **associated with hilar gland enlargement**, **pleural effusion**, areas of **collapse** or **consolidation**.
- **Cavitation found in 15%** (central air lucency, an air–fluid level and a wall of variable thickness). Squamous cell carcinomas frequently cavitate.
- May see **metastases**.

> **Note:** Alveolar cell carcinoma may present as widespread pulmonary shadowing rather than as a solitary mass.

Chest X-rays for Medical Students, First Edition. Christopher Clarke, Anthony Dux.
© 2011 John Wiley & Sons, Ltd. Published 2011 by Blackwell Publishing Ltd.

Heart failure

Heart failure is a syndrome defined as the **failure of the heart** to **maintain an adequate flow of blood to the tissues**.

There are many different causes of heart failure but the four main causes are:

1. ischaemic heart disease
2. non-ischaemic dilated cardiomyopathy
3. hypertension
4. valvular heart disease.

Radiological features associated with heart failure

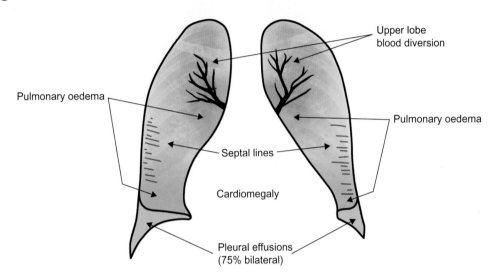

Figure 128 Radiological features of heart failure.

1. **Cardiomegaly** (*see* p. 72).
2. **Pulmonary oedema** (pink) (*see* p. 65)
   - +/– the atypical **'bat's wing' pattern shadowing** (*see* p. 67).
3. **Upper lobe blood diversion** (black)
   - vessels in upper lobes appear larger than vessels in the lower lobes on an erect chest X-ray due to increased pulmonary vascular resistance in the lower zones due to dependent oedema.
4. **Septal lines** (grey) (*see* p. 69)
   - due to fluid in the lymphatics.
5. **Pleural effusions** (green) (*see* p. 60)
   - fluid leaks from the vessels into the pleural space.

Example 1

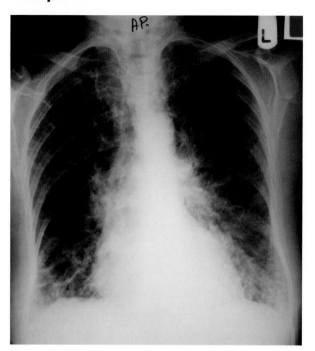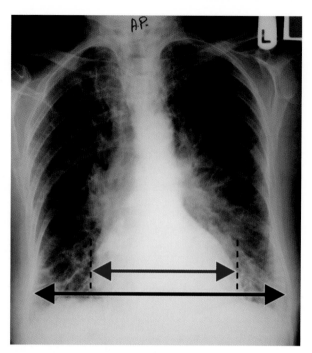

Figure 129 Two identical PA chest radiographs showing heart failure. The right radiograph shows pulmonary oedema marked in pink and septal lines marked in yellow. The black dotted lines mark the edge of the heart. The shorter red arrow marks the width of the heart. The longer black arrow marks the width of the thoracic cavity. The width of the heart is greater than half the width of the thoracic cavity, therefore there is also cardiomegaly.

Example 2

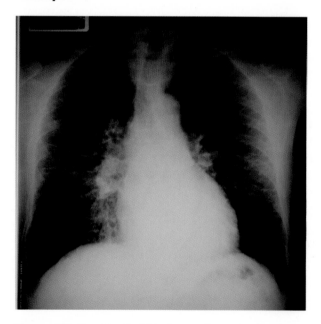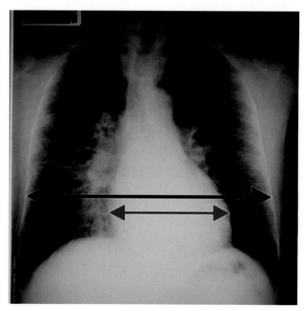

Figure 130 Two identical PA chest radiographs showing congestive heart failure. The right radiograph shows pulmonary oedema marked in pink and septal lines marked in yellow. The black dotted lines mark the edge of the heart. The shorter red arrow marks the width of the heart. The longer black arrow marks the width of the thoracic cavity. The width of the heart is greater than half the width of the thoracic cavity, therefore there is also cardiomegaly.

Pneumonia

Pneumonia is **inflammation** of the **lung parenchyma** characterised by **filling of the alveoli air spaces** with **exudate** and **inflammatory cells**. On a chest X-ray pneumonia appears as **consolidation/airspace shadowing** (*see* p. 23).

Note: Consolidation and pneumonia are not the same thing and the terms should not be used interchangeably. Consolidation refers to any pathological process that involves the replacement of alveolar air by fluid, cells, pus or other material. That said, pneumonia is by far the most common cause of consolidation.

Types of pneumonia
- Community-acquired pneumonia   } Bacterial or viral infection
- Hospital-acquired pneumonia
- Aspiration pneumonia   } Inhalation of oropharyngeal secretions.

Other occasional features of pneumonia on a chest radiograph include:
- air bronchogram
- pleural effusion (parapneumonic effusion)
- cavitation.

Chronic obstructive pulmonary disease

Note: Chronic obstructive pulmonary disease (COPD) *cannot be diagnosed* from a chest X-ray. Always confirm COPD from the patient's clinical history and lung function tests.

If COPD is suspected look for the following.
- **Pneumothorax**
  - common in COPD so look for these (they can 'hide' in the lung apexes).
- **Mass lesion/metastasis/other signs of lung cancer**
  - a history of smoking is almost universal in COPD so look for evidence of bronchial carcinoma.

Tuberculosis

Tuberculosis (TB) is an infection most often caused by *Mycobacterium tuberculosis*, affecting mainly the respiratory tract, though it can involve any system in the body. Patients prone to infection are the **immunosuppressed**, **debilitated** and **immigrant populations**.

Tuberculosis has various manifestations in the lung and often presents in the lung **apices**.

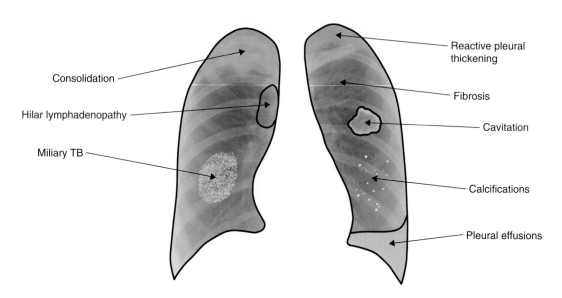

Figure 131 Radiological features of tuberculosis.

There is a lot of crossover between the radiological appearances of primary TB, secondary TB and previous (old) TB infection. Radiological appearances commonly associated with the different stages of TB are listed below.

- **Primary TB:**
  - peripheral lung mass/consolidation (Ghon focus)
  - enlarged hilar lymph nodes.
- **Secondary TB** (also known as **post-primary TB** or **reactive TB**):
  - consolidation often with cavitation
  - especially in upper lobes or apical segments of the lower lobes
  - may be associated with pleural effusions and/or pleural thickening.
- **Previous (old) TB** (as healing progresses, features you may recognise are):
  - fibrosis and volume loss
  - calcified foci
  - pleural calcification
  - **tuberculoma** ◄

> *A tuberculoma is a localised granuloma with a well-defined margin, often containing calcification. They are roughly 2 cm in diameter and remain unchanged on serial CXR examinations.*

- **Miliary TB:**
  - discrete 1–2 mm nodules distributed evenly throughout the lung fields due to haematogenous spread.

Example 1

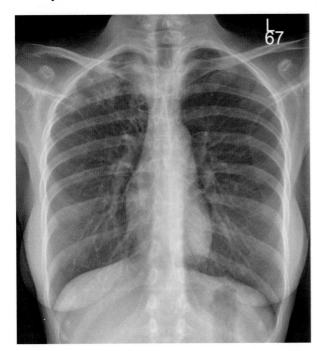
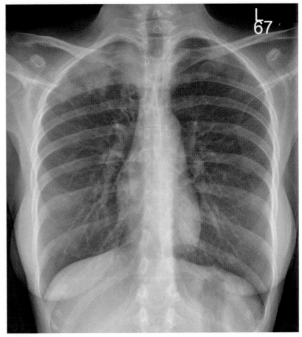

Figure 132 Two identical chest radiographs showing primary TB with right apical consolidation. There is patchy shadowing in the apex of the right lung. The right radiograph shows the consolidation of primary TB marked in green.

Example 2

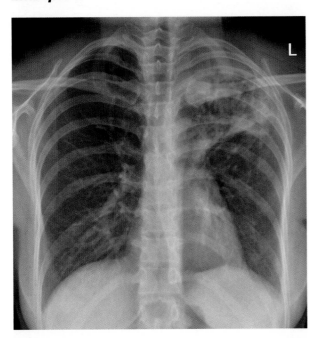
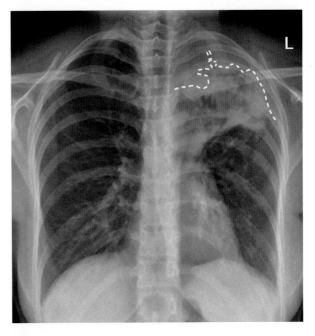

Figure 133 Two identical chest radiographs showing primary TB at the left apex. There is pleural thickening at the left apex seen as a homogenous shadow extending inwards from the edge of the thoracic cavity – this is likely to be reactive from the TB. There is left upper lobe consolidation with volume loss and some fibrotic change seen as patchy shadowing (consolidation) mixed with some reticulonodular shadowing (fibrosis). The right radiograph shows the pleural thickening marked in green superiorly and the consolidation/fibrosis marked in green inferiorly. A dotted white line separates the pleural thickening (above) from the consolidation/fibrosis (below).

Example 3

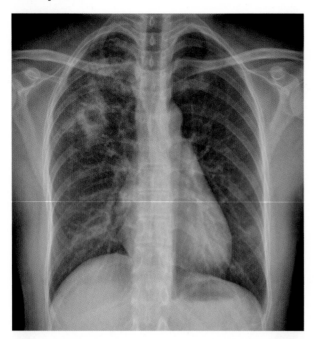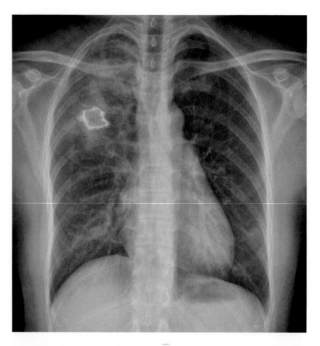

Figure 134 Two identical chest radiographs showing primary TB with right upper lobe consolidation and cavity formation. There is patchy shadowing in the right upper lobe. The right radiograph shows the consolidation of primary TB marked in green, the cavity marked in yellow and the wall of the cavity marked in pale yellow.

Example 4

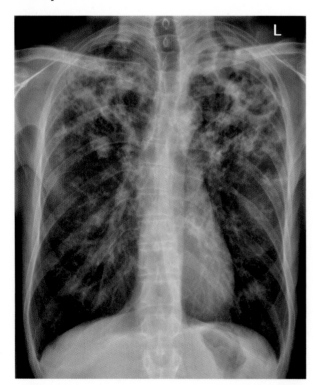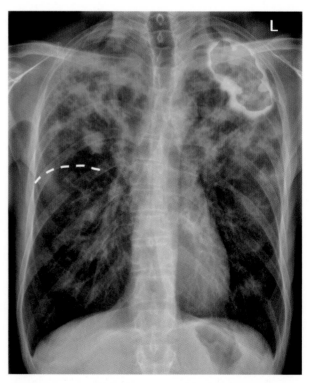

Figure 135 Two identical chest radiographs showing primary TB with bilateral upper lobe consolidation and cavity formation. There is patchy shadowing in both upper lobes. We know this is consolidation rather than fibrosis as there is no volume loss. If you look closely you can see that the horizontal fissure is not deviated upwards. The right radiograph shows the consolidation of primary TB marked in green, the cavity marked in yellow, the wall of the cavity marked in pale yellow and the horizontal fissure marked with a white dotted line.

Example 5

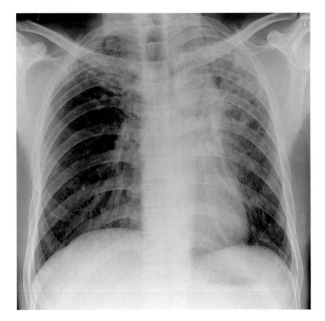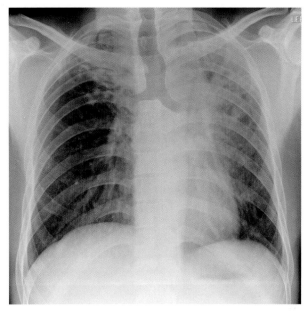

Figure 136 Two identical chest radiographs showing secondary TB (reactivation) with left upper lobe volume loss, left hilar lymph node enlargement and pervious (old) TB changes in the right upper lobe. There is patchy shadowing in both upper lobes. There is elevation of the left hilum, and the left main bronchus is pulled superiorly, causing widening of the carinal angle. The right radiograph shows the consolidation/fibrosis of secondary TB marked in green, the enlarged hilar lymph node marked in orange and the trachea/left main bronchus/right main bronchus marked in blue.

Example 6

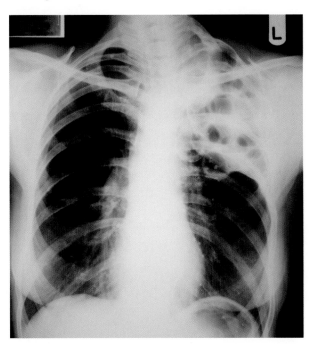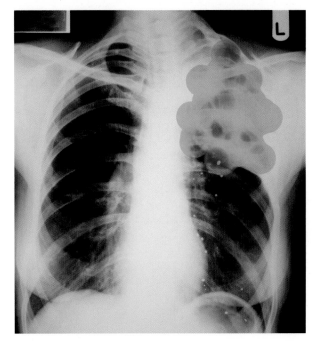

Figure 137 Two identical chest radiographs showing old TB in a patient who had a thoracoplasty and plombage due to previous TB infection. Plombage was a surgical method used before the introduction of TB antibiotics to treat TB of the upper lobe of the lung. The term derives from the French word *'plomb'* (lead) and refers to the insertion of an inert substance into the pleural space, the theory being that if the diseased lobe of the lung was physically forced to collapse, it would heal more quickly. You can see the plombage in the left upper zone and also some calcified foci in the left lung. The right radiograph shows the plombage marked in pink and the calcified foci marked in yellow.

Examples 7, 8 & 9

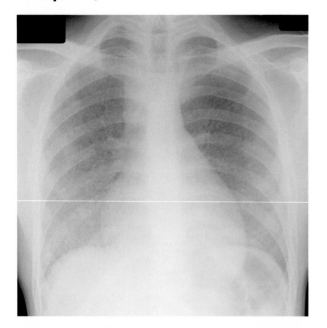

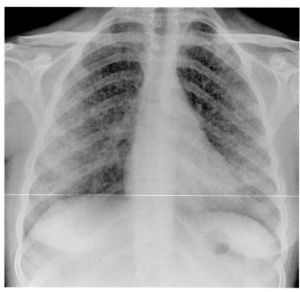

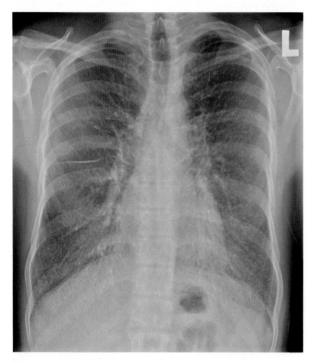

Figure 138 (top left) A chest radiograph showing miliary TB throughout both lungs. There are discrete 1–2 mm nodules distributed evenly throughout the lung fields.

Figure 139 (top right) A chest radiograph showing miliary TB throughout both lungs. There are discrete 1–2 mm nodules distributed evenly throughout the lung fields.

Figure 140 (bottom left) A chest radiograph showing miliary TB throughout both lungs. There are discrete 1–2 mm nodules distributed evenly throughout the lung fields.

Asbestos-related lung disease

Inhalation of **asbestos fibres** is an industrial hazard that can lead to chest disease. Patients may be entitled to compensation as it is considered to be an occupational lung disease. The incidence of bronchial carcinoma in people who have worked with asbestos is five times higher in non-smokers and 50 times higher in smokers.

There are three disease categories:

1. **benign pleural disease**
2. **asbestosis**
3. **mesothelioma**.

Benign pleural disease

The distinctive radiological features are **asbestos plaques**. Asbestos plaques are **pleural plaques – areas of pleural thickening** caused by **asbestos fibres**. They give a localised area of whiteness on a CXR. Patients may also develop pleural effusions.

Radiological features

- **Pleural plaques** are *irregular opacities* with *well-defined edges*. They are commonly found running *along the line of the anterior ribs* and are usually *bilateral*. Often they can have *areas of patchy calcification within* them.
- **Calcified pleural plaques** may be found running *along the diaphragm*.
- **Diffuse pleural thickening** that appears as a thickened line around the edge of the lung.
- **Pleural effusions** may develop after a latent period averaging 10 years after exposure.

> **Note:** Compare to an old X-ray. Pleural plaques are slow growing and are probably visible on a previous X-ray.

Example 1

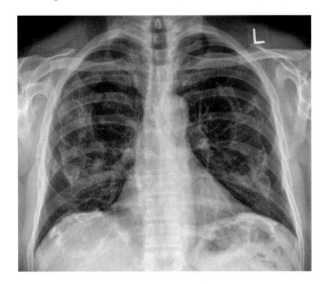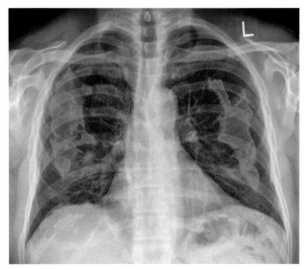

Figure 141 Two identical chest radiographs showing two large pleural plaques, one in each lung. Note the well-defined edges and the areas of patchy calcification (whiteness) within. There are also calcified pleural plaques running along the diaphragm. The right radiograph shows the pleural plaques marked in green.

Example 2

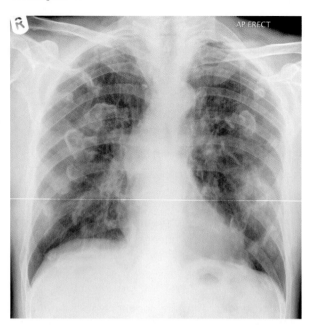 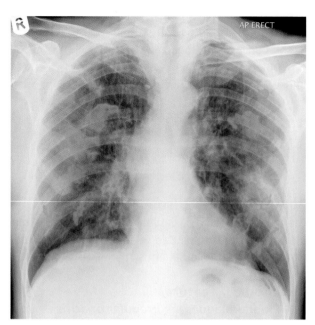

Figure 142 Two identical chest radiographs showing multiple pleural plaques throughout both lung fields. Note the well-defined edges and the areas of patchy calcification (whiteness) within. The right radiograph shows the pleural plaques marked in green.

Asbestosis

Asbestosis is the term for the **interstitial fibrosis** that develops in approximately 50% of patients with industrial asbestos exposure. It is a **chronic inflammatory condition** affecting the **interstitial tissue** of the lungs, occurring after long-term, heavy exposure to asbestos (e.g. mining).

Radiological features
- **Fibrosis** with some **volume loss** (*see* Fibrosis, p. 49 for examples).
  AND
- **Pleural calcification**. Areas of patchy calcification, seen relating to the diaphragm and along the anterior chest wall.

Mesothelioma

- A mesothelioma is a **malignant tumour** that develops in the **pleura**, usually unilaterally and causes pleuritic type chest pain.
- **5–10%** of asbestos workers develop malignant mesothelioma.
- It has a **latent period of 20–45 years**.

1. Pleura
2. Mesothelioma

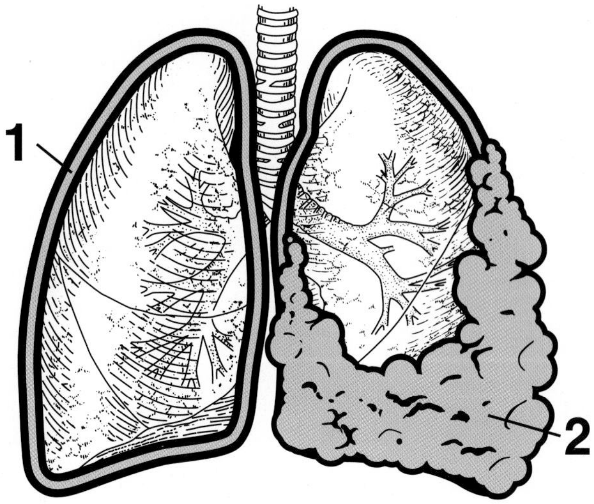

Figure 143 Diagrammatic representation of a left-sided mesothelioma. The pleural space is shown in green and you can see that the mesothelioma easily spreads within the pleural space encasing the lung. **1** Pleura. **2** Mesothelioma.

On a CXR, it gives characteristics of **pleural shadowing** (from diffuse, progressive thickening of the pleura and associated malignant pleural effusion) and evidence of **chest wall invasion** (metastasis).

Radiological features

- The spread of **whiteness does *not* follow lung lobe boundaries** as it is pleural in origin.
- The **edges** of the whiteness are **lobular** in nature *(suggests malignancy)*.
  - Look at the upper edges of the whiteness. There should be **no meniscus** (*this is because the main differential diagnosis to rule out is a pleural effusion*).
- There may be **loss of lung volume** on the affected side *(increases suspicion of mesothelioma)*.
- Evidence of chest wall invasion (**rib destruction** or **soft tissue mass in chest wall**) may be the only feature to differentiate mesothelioma from benign disease.

Note: Pleural tumours could be due to mesothelioma, other secondaries, benign tumours (rare) or pleural sarcoma (very rare).

Example 1

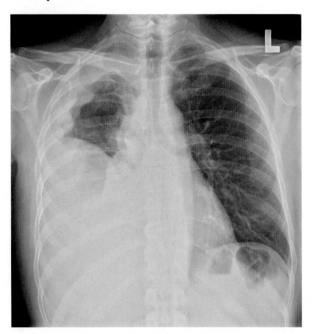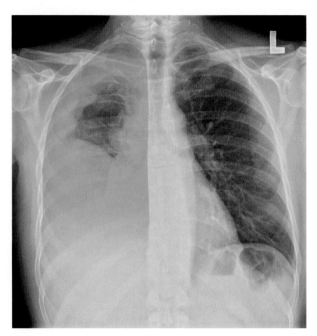

Figure 144 Two identical chest radiographs showing a large right-sided malignant mesothelioma. Note that the whiteness surrounds the whole right thoracic cavity, is lobular in nature and does not follow lung boundaries. The right radiograph shows the malignant mesothelioma marked in green.

Example 2

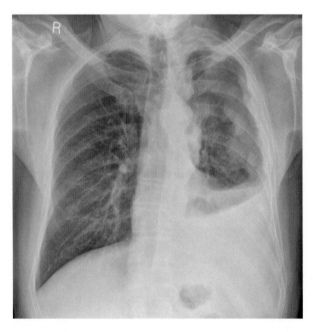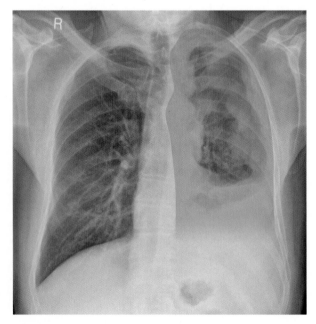

Figure 145 Two identical chest radiographs showing a large left-sided malignant mesothelioma. Note that the whiteness surrounds the whole left thoracic cavity, is lobular in nature and does not follow lung boundaries. There is also an associated left pleural effusion. The right radiograph shows the malignant mesothelioma and pleural effusion marked in green.

Example 3

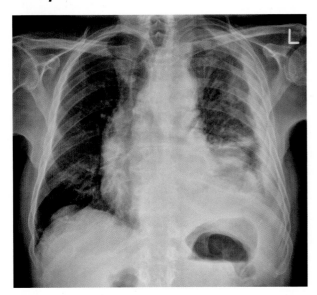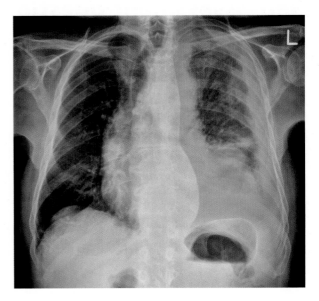

Figure 146 Two identical chest radiographs showing a large left-sided malignant mesothelioma. Note that the whiteness surrounds the whole left thoracic cavity, is lobular in nature and does not follow lung boundaries. The right radiograph shows the malignant mesothelioma marked in green.

Self-assessment questions

These questions test your ability to present a chest X-ray and recognise pathology. They are presented in the same format as an objective structured clinical examination (OSCE) or viva station, so to make it as real as possible there are no multiple-choice questions (MCQs).

There are 18 questions, each based on one chest X-ray. Remember to use the ABCDE approach when presenting and remember there may be **more than one pathology** in a single radiograph.

Part (a) of each question tests your ability to correctly present the X-ray using the ABCDE method and at the same time recognise pathology.

Parts (b), (c) and (d) are typical questions you may get asked in an OSCE and do not necessarily test facts learnt from this book. They are designed to test/teach you more general knowledge relating to the patient's pathology.

The answers can be found on pages 113–121.

Note: Any initials, ages and dates used are purely fictitious and are not related to the patient's X-ray in question.

Question 1

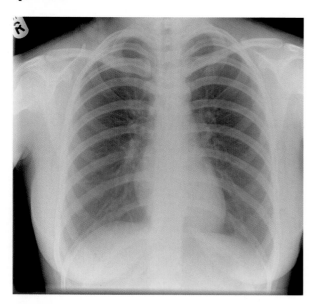

Figure 147 Name: Mrs LA, Age: 50. Date taken: 24/12/2011.
(a) Present this radiograph.
(b) Where is the anterior part of the left 2nd rib?
(c) Where is the border of the right atrium?
(d) Why is the right ventricle not visible on this radiograph?

Question 2

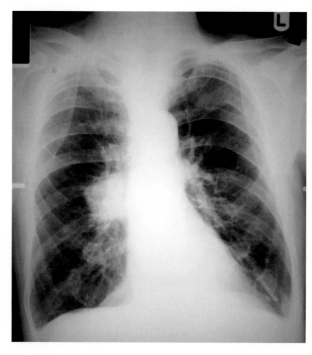

Figure 148 Name: Mr KH, Age: 60. Date taken: 27/07/2011.
(a) Present this radiograph.
(b) What is the most appropriate investigation to do next?

Question 3

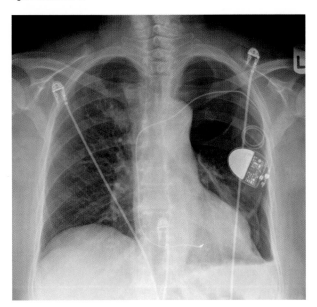

Figure 149 Name: Mrs HA, Age: 55. Date taken: 01/07/2011.

(a) Present this radiograph.

(b) What is the likely cause of this patient's pathology?

(c) If this was the first time you saw this, what would be the next step in this patient's management?

(d) What is the 'triangle of safety'?

Question 4

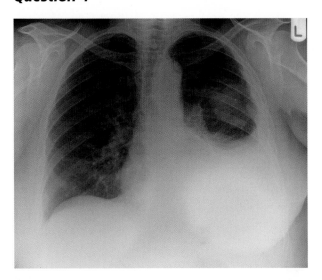

Figure 150 Name: Mrs NM, Age: 60. Date taken: 20/03/2011. Patient presented with dyspnoea.

(a) Present this radiograph.

(b) What is the likely cause of the abnormality in the lower zone of the left lung?

(c) Other than a staging CT scan, what would be the next step in this patient's management and what tests would you specifically send for?

Question 5

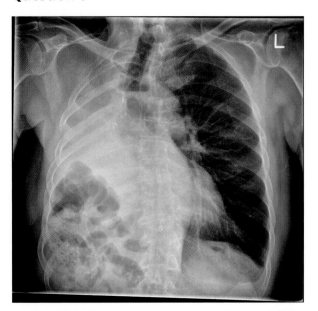

Figure 151 Name: Mr JS, Age: 70. Date taken: 11/02/2011.

(a) Present this radiograph.

(b) Why is this not just a pleural effusion?

(c) Why is this not lung collapse?

Question 6

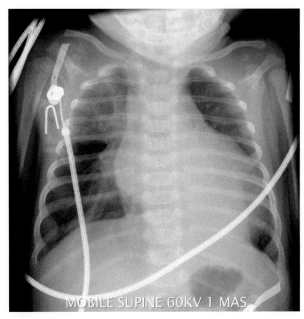

Figure 152 Name: Child NC, Age: 12 months. Date taken: 27/09/2011.

(a) Present this radiograph.

(b) Why do children collapse lobes or segments easily?

Question 7

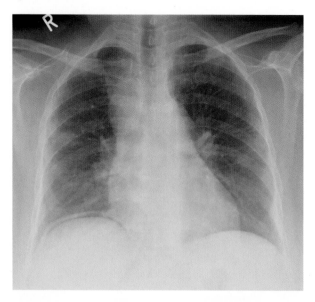

Figure 153 Name: Mrs DR, Age: 60. Date taken: 26/08/2011.
(a) Present this radiograph.
(b) The patient is complaining of severe abdominal pain. Given this radiograph, give four possible causes for this patient's pain.
(c) What are the causes for unilateral hilar lymphadenopathy?

Question 8

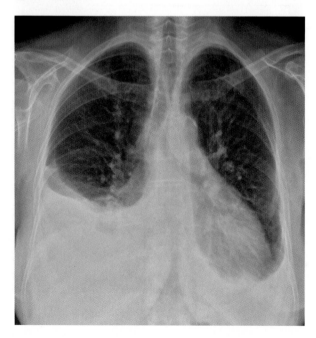

Figure 154 Name: Mrs ES, Age: 56. Date taken: 03/04/2011.
(a) Present this radiograph.
(b) Give three causes for pleural effusions.
(c) How might you distinguish between them?

Question 9

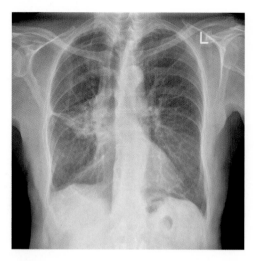

Figure 155 Name: Mr RR, Age: 61. Date taken: 12/02/2011.
(a) Present this radiograph.
(b) What is the diagnosis?
(c) Why has the middle lobe collapsed?

Question 10

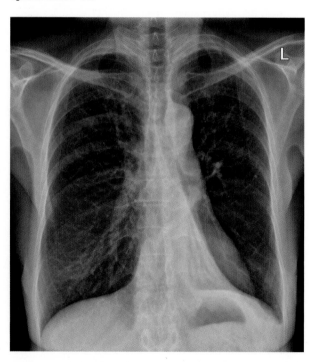

Figure 156 Name: Mrs WC, Age: 52. Date taken: 23/07/2011.
(a) Present this radiograph.
(b) What is the diagnosis?
(c) What follow-up would you recommend?

Question 11

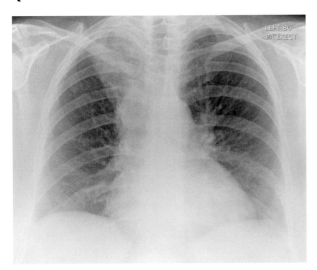

Figure 157 Name: Mr DC, Age: 38. Date taken: 11/12/2011.
(a) Present this radiograph.
(b) Give two possible causes for the abnormality in the right lung.
(c) What further investigation would you recommend? Please explain your answer?

Question 12

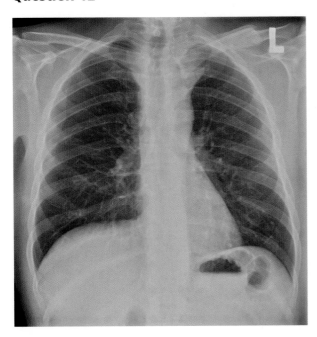

Figure 158 Name: Mrs MB, Age: 48. Date taken: 29/08/2011.
(a) Present this radiograph.
(b) What is the usual management of a clavicular fracture?
(c) What occasional chest complication may accompany a fractured clavicle?

Question 13

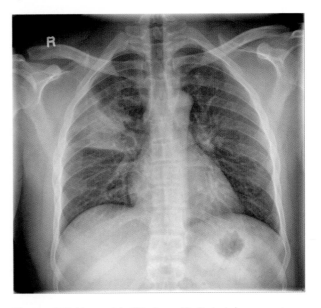

Figure 159 Name: Mr GB, Age: 43. Date taken: 02/08/2011.
(a) Present this radiograph.
(b) What is the diagnosis?
(c) What follow-up/further investigations would you recommend?

Question 14

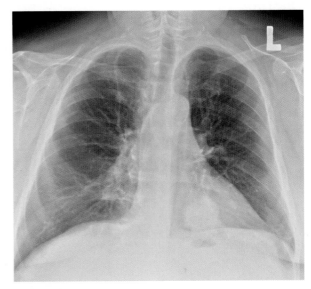

Figure 160 Name: Mr WC, Age: 71. Date taken: 08/10/2011.
(a) Present this radiograph.
(b) What is the likely differential diagnosis?
(c) What further investigation might you perform?

Question 15

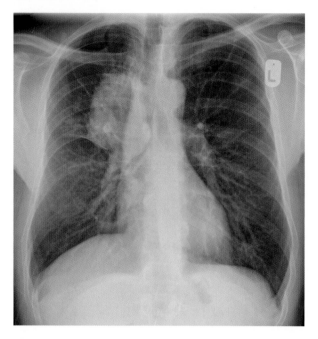

Figure 161 Name: Mr AC, Age: 62. Date taken: 30/08/2011.
(a) Present this radiograph.
(b) What is the likely diagnosis?
(c) What is the next investigation?

Question 16

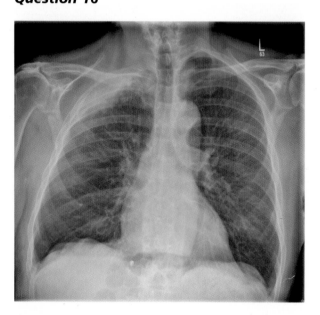

Figure 162 Name: Mr MF, Age: 67. Date taken: 06/03/2011.
(a) Present this radiograph.
(b) What is the likely diagnosis?
(c) What syndromes may be associated with this appearance?

Question 17

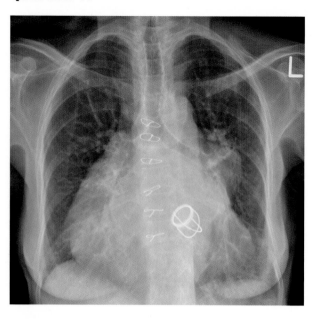

Figure 163 Name: Mrs MA, Age: 49. Date taken: 14/03/2011.
(a) Present this radiograph.
(b) How may this patient have presented clinically?
(c) What medication will this patient need for life?
(d) Why is there widening of the carinal angle?

Question 18

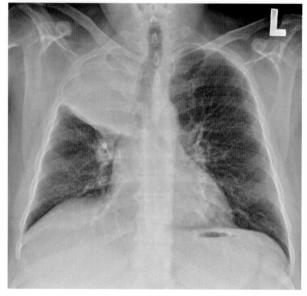

Figure 164 Name: Mr BW, Age: 64. Date taken: 30/05/2011.
(a) Present this radiograph.
(b) What is the diagnosis?
(c) In this particular radiograph, what is the likely cause of the abnormality identified?

Self-assessment answers

Answer 1

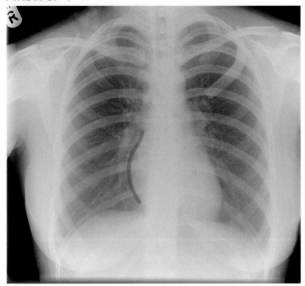

Figure 165 Name: Mrs LA, Age: 50. Date taken: 24/12/2011.

(a) This is a PA chest radiograph of Mrs LA, taken on 24 December 2011.
The film is not rotated and there is adequate inspiration.
A: The trachea is central.
B: The lungs are uniformly expanded and the lung fields are clear.
C: The heart size is normal. There is no mediastinal shift. The mediastinal contours and hila appear normal.
D: There is no fracture or bony abnormality.
E: There is no evidence of air under the diaphragm, surgical emphysema or any foreign body.
In summary, this is a normal chest radiograph.
(b) The anterior part of the left 2nd rib is marked in yellow.
(c) The border of the right atrium is the right heart border. It is marked in red.
(d) The right ventricle is not visible as it lies anteriorly and so does not have a border on a PA chest X-ray.

Answer 2

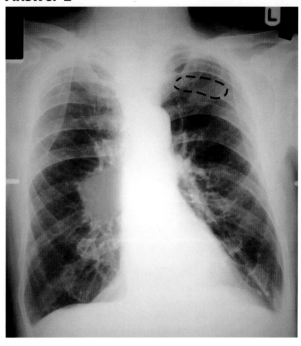

Figure 166 Name: Mr KH, Age: 60. Date taken: 27/07/2011.

(a) This is a PA chest radiograph of Mr KH, taken on 27 July 2011.
The film is not rotated and there is adequate inspiration.
A: The trachea is central.
B: The lungs are uniformly expanded and over-inflated. There is a large mass lesion with an irregular margin in the right mid-zone highly suggestive of malignancy (marked in red).
C: The heart size is normal. There is no mediastinal shift. The mediastinal contours and hila seem normal. I can see the border of the right hilum superimposed on the mass, therefore I know there is air between the mass and the right hilum, indicating that the mass is either anterior or posterior to the hilum, but not within the hilum.
D: There is a discontinuity in the posterior part of the left 5th rib (marked with a black dotted line), most likely caused by a bony metastasis.
E: There is no evidence of air under the diaphragm, surgical emphysema or any foreign body.
In summary, this is an abnormal chest radiograph, highly suggestive of a bronchial carcinoma with metastasis to the left 5th rib posteriorly.
(b) Staging CT of chest, abdomen and pelvis to look for metastasis and stage the cancer.

Chest X-rays for Medical Students, First Edition. Christopher Clarke, Anthony Dux.
© 2011 John Wiley & Sons, Ltd. Published 2011 by Blackwell Publishing Ltd.

Answer 3

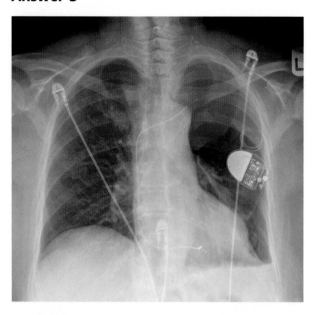

Figure 167 Name: Mrs HA, Age: 55. Date taken: 01/07/2011. Patient admitted with a history of collapse and a pacemaker was inserted. This X-ray was taken prior to discharge.

(a) This is a PA chest radiograph of Mrs HA, taken on 1 July 2011.
   The film is not rotated and there is adequate inspiration.
   A: The trachea is central.
   B: There is a left-sided pneumothorax (marked in blue). The lung edge is seen on the left side and there are no lung markings beyond the lung edge. Otherwise the lung fields are clear.
   C: The heart size is normal. There is no mediastinal shift. The mediastinal contours and hila appear normal.
   D: There is no fracture or bony abnormality.
   E: There is a cardiac pacemaker in situ and three ECG leads. There is no evidence of air under the diaphragm, surgical emphysema or any foreign body.
   In summary, this is an abnormal chest radiograph in a patient with a cardiac pacemaker as there is a left-sided pneumothorax.
(b) Pneumothorax secondary to pacemaker insertion.
(c) Insert a chest drain (with an underwater seal) into the pleural space.
(d) The area between the anterior axillary (1) and mid-axillary (2) lines and an imaginary horizontal line at the level of the nipples (3). This is the safe area to insert a chest drain (see Figure 168).

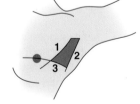

Figure 168

Answer 4

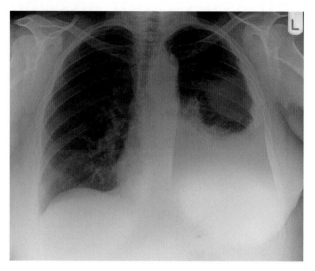

Figure 169 Name: Mrs NM, Age: 60. Date taken: 20/03/2011. Patient presented with dyspnoea.

(a) This is a PA chest radiograph of Mrs NM, taken on 20 March 2011.
   The film is not rotated and there is adequate inspiration.
   A: The trachea is central.
   B: There is a left-sided pleural effusion (marked in green). This is shown by a homogenous, dense opacity in the left lower zone with loss of the left costophrenic angle and hemidiaphragm. The upper edge is concave in shape and a meniscus is seen laterally.
   There is also a large mass lesion in the left mid-zone highly suggestive of malignancy (marked in red).
   C: The heart size is difficult to assess accurately as the left heart border is hidden by the pleural effusion. There is no mediastinal shift. The mediastinal contours and hila appear normal.
   D: There is no fracture or bony abnormality.
   E: There is no evidence of air under the diaphragm, surgical emphysema or any foreign body.
   In summary, this is an abnormal chest radiograph showing a left-sided pleural effusion and a left-sided mass lesion, highly suggestive of a bronchial carcinoma.
(b) The pleural effusion is most likely a malignant pleural effusion secondary to a bronchial carcinoma.
(c) The next step in this patient's management would be to obtain a sample of pleural fluid by performing an ultrasound-guided pleural aspirate. This should be sent to:
   • cytology – to look for malignant cells
   • biochemistry – to determine protein content to see if the fluid is an exudate or transudate
   • microbiology – to culture the fluid for infective organisms and determine antibiotic sensitivities.

Answer 5

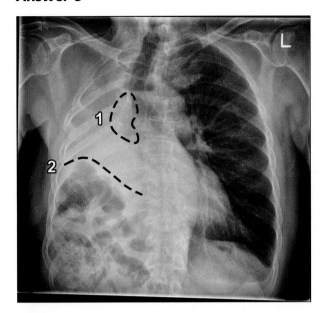

Figure 170 Name: Mr JS, Age: 70. Date taken: 11/02/2011.

(a) This is a PA chest radiograph of Mr JS, taken on 11 February 2011.
   The film is not rotated and there is adequate inspiration.
   A: The trachea is deviated to the right (marked in blue).
   B: There is evidence of a previous right pneumonectomy and associated volume loss. There is diffuse haziness throughout the right hemithorax and surgical slips are seen in the right hilar region (1). Loops of bowel are seen in the right hemithorax, due to volume loss and associated superior displacement of the right hemidiaphragm (2). The left lung is over inflated.
   C: The heart size is difficult to assess accurately as the right heart border is hidden by the diffuse haziness. There is mediastinal shift to the right. The mediastinal contours and hila appear normal.
   D: There is no fracture or bony abnormality.
   E: There is no evidence of air under the diaphragm, surgical emphysema or any foreign body.
   In summary, this is an abnormal chest radiograph showing a previous right pneumonectomy.
(b) This is not a pleural effusion because the trachea is deviated to the right side indicating a loss of volume. With a pleural effusion the trachea is usually central or if massive, then the trachea may be pushed towards the opposite side.
(c) Unless there is evidence of a thoracotomy or previous surgery, it is difficult to differentiate between complete lung collapse and a pneumonectomy. However, we know this is a pneumonectomy, not lung collapse, because there are surgical clips (1) as evidence of previous surgery.

Answer 6

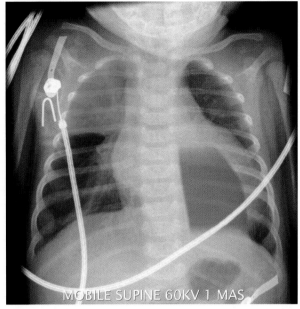

Figure 171 Name: Child NC, Age: 12 months. Date taken: 27/09/2011.

(a) This is an AP supine chest radiograph of Mr NC, taken on 27 September 2011.
   The film is not rotated and there is adequate inspiration.
   A: The trachea is central.
   B: The lungs are uniformly expanded and there is right upper lobe consolidation (marked in green). The patchy shadowing corresponds to the right upper lobe and there is no loss of lung volume. There is left lower lobe collapse (marked in blue). There is a triangular opacity behind the left heart shadow with loss of definition of the medial part of the left hemidiaphragm. The heart border is not obscured.
   C: I cannot comment on the heart size as this is an AP supine film. There is no mediastinal shift. The mediastinal contours and hila appear normal.
   D: There is no fracture or bony abnormality.
   E: There is no evidence of air under the diaphragm, surgical emphysema or any foreign body.
   In summary, this is an abnormal chest radiograph showing right upper lobe consolidation and left lower lobe collapse.
(b) The paediatric airways are narrow and become narrower as a result of inflammation. They then become obstructed by mucus plugs causing distal collapse and/or consolidation.

Answer 7

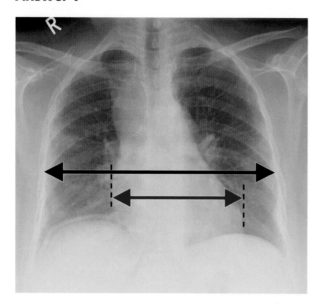

Figure 172 Name: Mrs DR, Age: 60. Date taken: 26/08/2011.

(a) This is a PA chest radiograph of Mrs DR, taken on 26 August 2011.

The film is not rotated and there is adequate inspiration.

A: The trachea is central.

B: The lungs are uniformly expanded.

C: There is cardiomegaly. The width of the heart is greater than half the width of the thoracic cavity (black dotted lines mark the edge of the heart, the shorter red arrow marks the width of the heart, the longer black arrow marks the width of the thoracic cavity). There is no mediastinal shift. There is a large shadow in the right upper mediastinum with a smooth lobular appearance consistent with right hilar lymph node enlargement (marked in orange).

D: There is no fracture or bony abnormality.

E: There is a rim of blackness beneath and very closely opposed to the curve of the right hemidiaphragm indicating air under the diaphragm (marked in blue). There is no surgical emphysema or any foreign body.

In summary, this is an abnormal chest radiograph showing cardiomegaly, right hilar lymph node enlargement and pneumoperitoneum.

(b) Possible causes of abdominal pain with a pneumoperitoneum are perforated peptic ulcer, perforated hollow viscus, air in the abdomen post-surgery and trauma.

(c) Causes of unilateral hilar lymphadenopathy are infection (e.g. TB), spread from a primary lung tumour or a primary lymphoma. Sarcoidosis is another possible cause; however, it is rarely unilateral.

Answer 8

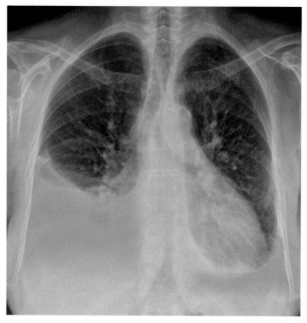

Figure 173 Name: Mrs ES, Age: 56. Date taken: 03/04/2011.

(a) This is a PA chest radiograph of Mrs ES, taken on 3 April 2011.

The film is not rotated and there is adequate inspiration.

A: The trachea is central.

B: There are bilateral pleural effusions. The right-sided effusion is larger than the left (marked in green). This is shown by a homogenous, dense opacity in both lower zones with loss of the costophrenic angles and hemidiaphragms. The upper edges are concave in shape and menisci are seen laterally.

C: The heart size is difficult to assess accurately as the right heart border is hidden by the pleural effusion. There is no mediastinal shift. The mediastinal contours and hila appear normal.

D: There is no fracture or bony abnormality.

E: There is no evidence of air under the diaphragm, surgical emphysema or any foreign body.

In summary, this is an abnormal chest radiograph showing bilateral pleural effusions.

(b) Heart failure, liver failure, renal failure.

(c) **1.** Heart failure: ECG and echocardiogram – to see if there is cardiac dysfunction.

2. Liver failure: liver biochemistry – to see if there is low serum albumin.

3. Renal failure: renal function – looking for raised creatinine and sodium/potassium imbalance.

Answer 9

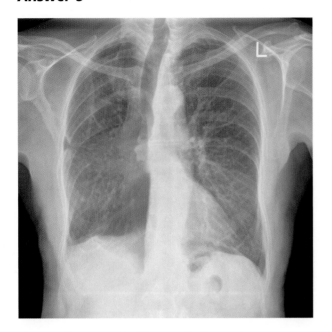

Figure 174 Name: Mr RR, Age: 61. Date taken: 12/02/2011.

(a) This is a PA chest radiograph of Mr RR, taken on 12 February 2011.
    The film is not rotated and there is adequate inspiration.
    A: The trachea is deviated to the right (marked in blue).
    B: The lungs are uniformly expanded. There is a large mass lesion in the right mid-zone, which may involve the hilum, highly suggestive of malignancy (marked in red).
    There is also middle lobe collapse (marked in blue). There is an increased density in the right mid-zone and the right heart border is obscured.
    C: The heart size is normal. There is no mediastinal shift. The left mediastinal contour appears normal.
    D: There is no fracture or bony abnormality.
    E: There is no evidence of air under the diaphragm, surgical emphysema or any foreign body.
    In summary, this is an abnormal chest radiograph showing right tracheal deviation, middle lobe collapse and a right-sided mass lesion highly suggestive of a bronchial carcinoma.
(b) Bronchial carcinoma and middle lobe collapse.
(c) It is likely the middle lobe has collapsed secondary to the mass lesion compressing and obstructing the middle lobe bronchus.

Answer 10

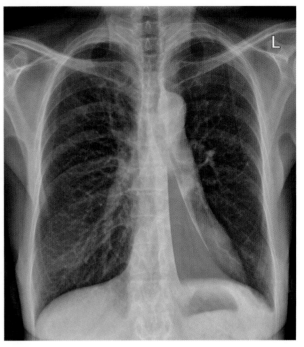

Figure 175 Name: Mrs WC, Age: 52. Date taken: 23/07/2011.

(a) This is a PA chest radiograph of Mrs WC, taken on 23 July 2011.
    The film is not rotated and there is adequate inspiration.
    A: The trachea is central.
    B: The lungs are uniformly expanded. There is left lower lobe collapse (marked in blue). There is a triangular opacity behind the left heart shadow and the left heart border is not obscured.
    C: The heart size is normal. There is no mediastinal shift. The mediastinal contours and hila appear normal.
    D: There is no fracture or bony abnormality.
    E: There is no evidence of air under the diaphragm, surgical emphysema or any foreign body.
    In summary, this is an abnormal chest radiograph showing left lower lobe collapse.
(b) Left lower lobe collapse.
(c) The main differential diagnosis is collapse secondary to infection; however, bronchial obstruction due to a bronchial carcinoma can also cause collapse. For follow-up a repeat X-ray is recommended in 4–6 weeks to look for any underlying malignancy.

Answer 11

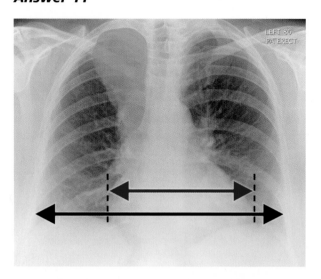

Figure 176 Name: Mr DC, Age: 38. Date taken: 11/12/2011.

(a) This is a PA chest radiograph of Mr DC, taken on 11 December 2011.
The film is not rotated and there is adequate inspiration.
A: The trachea is central.
B: The lungs are uniformly expanded and there is right upper lobe collapse/consolidation (marked in green). The patchy shadowing corresponds to the right upper lobe and the horizontal fissure is pulled upwards, indicating a loss of upper lobe volume.
C: There is cardiomegaly. The width of the heart is greater than half the width of the thoracic cavity (black dotted lines mark the edge of the heart, the shorter red arrow marks the width of the heart, the longer black arrow marks the width of the thoracic cavity). There is no mediastinal shift. There is a large shadow in the right upper mediastinum with a smooth lobular appearance consistent with right paratracheal lymph node enlargement (marked in orange).
D: There is no fracture or bony abnormality.
E: There is no evidence of air under the diaphragm, surgical emphysema or any foreign body.
In summary, this is an abnormal chest radiograph showing right upper lobe collapse/consolidation, right paratracheal lymph node enlargement and cardiomegaly.
(b) (1) Pneumonia; (2) possible underlying malignancy.
(c) There are three possible answers.
1. Follow up chest X-ray – to see if the collapse/ consolidation and enlarged lymph node had resolved.
2. Bronchoscopy – to look for bronchial narrowing (e.g. tumour).
3. CT chest – to look for a possible mass.

Answer 12

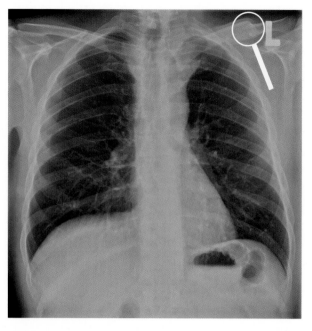

Figure 177 Name: Mrs MB, Age: 48. Date taken: 29/08/2011.

(a) This is a PA chest radiograph of Mrs MB, taken on 29 August 2011.
The film is not rotated and there is adequate inspiration.
A: The trachea is central.
B: The lungs are uniformly expanded and the lung fields are clear.
C: The heart size is normal. There is no mediastinal shift. The mediastinal contours and hila appear normal.
D: There is a fracture-dislocation of the left clavicle (marked by a white circle).
E: There is no evidence of air under the diaphragm, surgical emphysema or any foreign body.
In summary, this is an abnormal chest radiograph showing a fracture-dislocation of the left clavicle.
(b) The management is usually conservative with use of a 'collar and cuff' or similar support to take the weight of the arm off the clavicle.
(c) Pneumothorax.

Answer 13

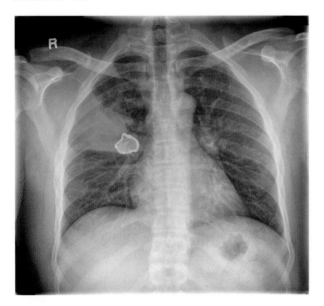

Figure 178 Name: Mr GB, Age: 43. Date taken: 02/08/2011.

(a) This is a PA chest radiograph of Mr GB, taken on 2 August 2011.
    The film is not rotated and there is adequate inspiration.
    A: The trachea is central.
    B: The lungs are uniformly expanded and there is a cavitating lung lesion in the right upper lobe (marked in yellow). It is associated with an area of consolidation fanning out from the cavity towards the edge of the lung (marked in green).
    C: The heart size is normal. There is no mediastinal shift. The mediastinal contours and hila appear normal.
    D: There is no fracture or bony abnormality.
    E: There is no evidence of air under the diaphragm, surgical emphysema or any foreign body.
    In summary, this is an abnormal chest radiograph showing a cavitating lung lesion in the right upper lobe with an associated area of consolidation.
(b) Lobar pneumonia with cavitation.
(c) Follow-up chest X-ray in 4–6 weeks to ensure resolution or reveal underlying mass lesion. Bronchoscopy should be performed if symptoms do not resolve or chest X-ray remains abnormal.

Answer 14

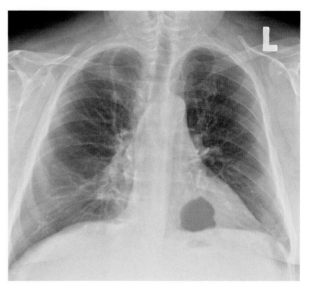

Figure 179 Name: Mr WC, Age: 71. Date taken: 08/10/2011.

(a) This is a PA chest radiograph of Mr WC, taken on 8 October 2011.
    The film is not rotated and there is adequate inspiration.
    A: The trachea is central.
    B: The lungs are uniformly expanded. There is a mass lesion in the left lower zone superimposed behind the heart shadow highly suggestive of malignancy (marked in red).
    C: The heart size is normal. There is no mediastinal shift. The mediastinal contours and hila appear normal.
    D: There is no fracture or bony abnormality.
    E: There is no evidence of air under the diaphragm, surgical emphysema or any foreign body.
    In summary, this is an abnormal chest radiograph showing a left-sided mass lesion highly suggestive of a bronchial carcinoma.
(b) Bronchial carcinoma or large solitary metastasis.
(c) CT of the thorax and possible biopsy. The CT field could include the kidneys as one of the possible causes of a large solitary metastasis is a renal carcinoma.

Answer 15

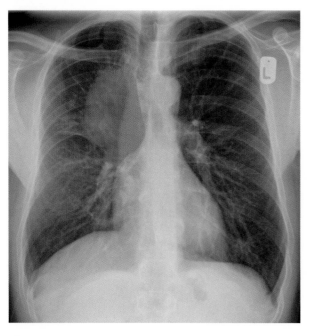

Figure 180 Name: Mr AC, Age: 62. Date taken: 30/08/2011.

(a) This is a PA chest radiograph of Mr AC, taken on 30 August 2011.
   The film is not rotated and there is adequate inspiration.
   A: The trachea is central.
   B: The lungs are uniformly expanded. There is a large mass lesion in the right upper zone compressing the right main bronchus, highly suggestive of malignancy (marked in red).
   C: The heart size is normal. There is no mediastinal shift. The mediastinal contours and hila appear normal.
   D: There is no fracture or bony abnormality.
   E: There is no evidence of air under the diaphragm, surgical emphysema or any foreign body.
   In summary, this is an abnormal chest radiograph showing a right-sided mass lesion highly suggestive of a bronchial carcinoma.
(b) A large central tumour.
(c) Bronchoscopy and trans-bronchial biopsy as the tumour is central. A CT scan may be performed subsequently as an aid to staging.

Answer 16

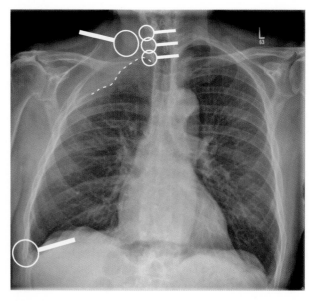

Figure 181 Name: Mr MF, Age: 67. Date taken: 06/03/2011.

(a) This is a PA chest radiograph of Mr MF, taken on 6 March 2011.
   The film is not rotated and there is adequate inspiration.
   A: The trachea is central.
   B: There is a mass lesion in the right apex (marked in red) with associated pleural thickening (marked in green).
   C: The heart size is normal. There is no mediastinal shift. The mediastinal contours and hila appear normal.
   D: There is complete lysis of the right 1st rib and erosions of the upper right transverse processes of the upper thoracic vertebrae. There is also a fracture of the right 9th rib (each marked by a white circle).
   E: There is no evidence of air under the diaphragm, surgical emphysema or any foreign body.
   In summary, this is an abnormal chest radiograph showing a right-sided apical mass lesion with associated pleural thickening and complete lysis of the right 1st rib, highly suggestive of a bronchial carcinoma. There is also a fracture of the right 9th rib, which may be coincidental.
(b) Right-sided Pancoast tumour.
(c) Horner's syndrome and Pancoast's syndrome.

Answer 17

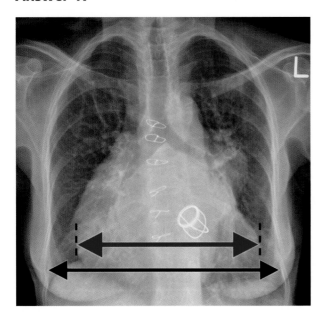

Figure 182 Name: Mrs MA, Age: 49. Date taken: 14/03/2011.

(a) This is a PA chest radiograph of Mrs MA, taken on 14 March 2011.
   The film is not rotated and there is adequate inspiration.

   A: The trachea is central. There is widening of the carinal angle (trachea and mainstem bronchi marked in blue).

   B: The lungs are uniformly expanded and the lung fields are clear.

   C: There is cardiomegaly. The width of the heart is greater than half the width of the thoracic cavity (black dotted lines mark the edge of the heart, the shorter red arrow marks the width of the heart, the longer black arrow marks the width of the thoracic cavity). The mediastinal contours and hila appear normal.

   D: There is no fracture or bony abnormality.

   E: There is a mechanical heart valve in situ and median sternotomy wires are noted. There is no evidence of air under the diaphragm, surgical emphysema or any foreign body.
   In summary, this is an abnormal chest radiograph showing widening of the carinal angle, cardiomegaly, a mechanical heart valve in situ and median sternotomy wires.

(b) Atrial fibrillation due to mitral valve disease.

(c) Lifetime anticoagulation.

(d) There is obviously mitral valve disease which causes left atrial enlargement. This will in turn cause widening of the carinal angle.

Answer 18

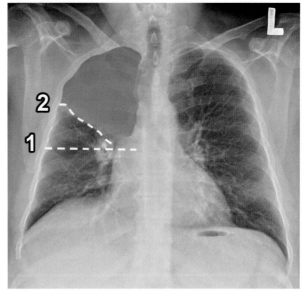

Figure 183 Name: Mr BW, Age: 64. Date taken: 30/05/2011.

(a) This is a PA chest radiograph of Mr BW, taken on 30 May 2011.
   The film is not rotated and there is adequate inspiration.

   A: The trachea is central.

   B: The lungs are uniformly expanded. There is right upper lobe collapse/consolidation (marked in blue). There is increased density of the right upper zone, elevation of the horizontal fissure and loss of definition of the upper right mediastinal margins (the position of the horizontal fissure in a normal lung is shown with white dotted line **1**. The abnormal position of the raised horizontal fissure in this radiograph is shown with white dotted line **2**).

   C: The heart size is normal. There is no mediastinal shift. The mediastinal contours and hila appear normal.

   D: There is no fracture or bony abnormality.

   E: There is no evidence of air under the diaphragm, surgical emphysema or any foreign body.
   In summary, this is an abnormal chest radiograph showing right upper lobe collapse/consolidation.

(b) Right upper lobe collapse/consolidation. This is not total collapse as the horizontal fissure is only marginally displaced and the upper lobe is opaque due to purulent infiltrates within the airspaces (consolidation).

(c) In this adult patient the most likely cause would be a central bronchial neoplasm causing narrowing of the upper lobe bronchus with consequent infection. A primary pneumonia remains a possibility and the clinical presentation should determine whether antibiotic treatment with radiological follow-up is a better option than referral for bronchosopy

Glossary

Abscess – a localised collection of pus surrounded by inflamed tissue

Aetiology – the cause of a disease

Air bronchogram – the radiographic appearance of an air-filled bronchus that is surrounded by fluid-filled or solid alveoli

Alveoli – tiny air sacs within the lungs where the exchange of oxygen and carbon dioxide takes place

Anterior – located in front of or towards the front of a structure

Anticoagulant – a substance that prevents the clotting of blood

AP (anterior–posterior) – the X-ray tube is placed in front of the patient and the X-rays pass in the anterior–posterior direction

Apex (of the lung) – meaning the tip of something, it refers to the most superior portion of the lung (*pleural: apices*)

Arteriovenous malformation – an abnormal connection between veins and arteries, usually congenital

Asbestos plaques – deposits of fibrous tissue that develop in the chest cavity as a result of asbestos exposure

Asbestosis – an irreversible chronic inflammatory condition affecting the parenchymal tissue of the lungs caused by the inhalation and retention of asbestos fibres. It is one of the causes of lung fibrosis

Ascending – moving towards a higher level or position

Aspirate – to suction or to inhale, e.g. fluid into the lungs after vomiting

Atelectasis – collapse of lung tissue affecting part or all of one lung

Attenuated – having undergone a process of attenuation (*see* **Attenuation**)

Attenuation – the process by which a beam of radiation is reduced in energy when passing through some material

Auscultation – the act of listening for sounds made by internal organs, such as the heart and lungs, to aid in the diagnosis of certain disorders, usually using a stethoscope

Axilla – analogous to the armpit (*pleural:* **axillae**)

'Bat's wing' pattern – the radiological appearance of bilateral or unilateral ill-defined opacities confined to the central (peri-hilar) area of the lungs, as seen in acute pulmonary oedema

Benign – not recurrent or progressive; not malignant

Bifurcation – where a structure splits or divides into two

Bilateral – involving both sides

Biochemistry – the laboratory department studying the chemical composition of a biological substance, e.g. protein content in a pleural fluid aspirate

Bronchial – relating to the bronchi (*see* **Bronchus**)

Bronchial breathing – breath sounds of a harsh or blowing quality, heard on auscultation of the chest, made by air moving in the large bronchi

Bronchiectasis – a persistent or progressive lung condition characterised by dilated thick-walled bronchi

Bronchogram – *see* **Air bronchogram**

Bronchoscopy – a technique for visualising the inside of the airways using a bronchoscope

Bronchus – a subdivision of the trachea serving to convey air to and from the lungs (*pleural:* **bronchi**)

Calcification – the process by which calcium builds up in soft tissues

Cannula – a hollow tube that is inserted into a body cavity, duct or vessel to drain or administer a substance

Carcinoma – a malignant tumour derived from epithelial tissue

Cardiomegaly – enlargement of the heart. If the width of the heart on a PA chest radiograph is more than half the total width of the thorax, then the patient has cardiomegaly

Cardiomyopathy – a disease or disorder of the heart muscle

Carina – the site of tracheal bifurcation

Carinal angle – the angle between the left and right mainstem bronchi

Cavitation – a hole in the lung with a wall, lumen and contents

Chronic obstructive pulmonary disease (COPD) – an umbrella term for the condition affecting people with chronic bronchitis, emphysema or both

Collapse – *see* **Atelectasis**

Computed tomography (CT) – a medical imaging technique that uses X-rays to produce an image of a detailed cross-section of tissue

Computed tomography pulmonary angiography (CTPA) – a diagnostic test using computed tomography (CT) to obtain an image of the pulmonary arteries. Its main use is to diagnose a pulmonary embolism (PE)

Concave – curving inwards

Concavity – *see* **Concave**

Connective tissue – stroma; a fibrous tissue of mesodermal origin supporting organs, filling the spaces between them and forming tendons and ligaments

Consolidation – also known as airspace shadowing, is the replacement of alveolar air by fluid, cells, pus or other material

Contrast – the difference in absorption between one tissue and another

COPD – *see* **Chronic obstructive pulmonary disease**

Costophrenic angle – the angle between the ribs and the diaphragm on a chest radiograph

Crepitation – a crackling sound made by tissue, caused by the presence of gas

CT – *see* **Computed tomography**

CTPA – *see* **Computed tomography pulmonary angiography**

CXR – abbreviation for chest X-ray

Cytology – the laboratory department studying cells, e.g. cell numbers and types in a pleural fluid aspirate

Density – the mass per unit volume

Dependent oedema – an abnormal accumulation of fluid in the intercellular spaces of the body that appears to be influenced by gravity

Diaphragm – the musculomembranous partition separating the thoracic and abdominal cavities and acting as the major muscle for inspiration

Diverticulum – an outpouching of a hollow or fluid-filled viscous, e.g. large bowel diverticulum

ECG (electrocardiography) – a test that records the electrical activity of the heart

ECMO – *see* **Extra corporeal membrane oxygenation**

Effusion – the escape of fluid into a tissue or cavity (e.g. from blood vessels or lymph into the pleural space)

Electromagnetic radiation – a form of energy exhibiting wave-like behaviour as it travels through space. It is classified according to the frequency of its wave

Electromagnetic spectrum – the range of all possible frequencies of electromagnetic radiation

Emphysema – an abnormal distension of body tissues caused by retention of air (*see also* **Chronic obstructive pulmonary disease** *and* **Subcutaneous emphysema**)

Endobronchial – within or passing through a bronchus

Endotracheal – within or passing through the trachea

Engorgement – distension of body tissues caused by vascular or lymph congestion

Erect – upright in position or posture

Expiration – breathing out

Exposure – the quantifiable dose of radiation on a subject

Extra corporeal membrane oxygenation – a life support system that circulates the blood through an oxygenating system, similar to a heart–lung bypass machine

Extrapulmonary – outside of the lungs

Extrinsic allergic alveolitis – diffuse inflammation of the lung parenchyma and airways in people who have been sensitised by repeated inhalation of organic antigens in dusts. One of the causes of lung fibrosis

Exudate – an extravascular fluid with high protein content (>30 g/l of protein)

Fibrosis – the formation or development of excess fibrous connective tissue in an organ or tissue as a reparative or reactive process, as opposed to a formation of fibrous tissue as a normal constituent of an organ or tissue (e.g. lung fibrosis)

Fissure – a natural deep cleft separating one lobe from another in the lungs and lined by visceral pleura

Foreign body – any object originating outside the body

Ghon focus – an area of granulomatous inflammation in the lung caused by tuberculosis in a previously unaffected individual

Gland – an aggregation of cells specialised to synthesise a substance for release such as hormones

Haemothorax – a condition that results from blood accumulating in the pleural cavity

Hamartoma – a benign tumour-like malformation resulting from faulty development in an organ and composed of an abnormal mixture of tissue elements that develop and grow at the same rate as normal elements but are not likely to compress adjacent tissue

Heart failure – an inability of the heart to maintain adequate blood circulation to the peripheral tissues and the lungs

Hemidiaphragm – half of the diaphragm, the muscle that separates the chest cavity from the abdomen and that serves as the main muscle of respiration

Hemithorax – one side of the chest

Hiatus hernia – herniation of the stomach into the thorax

Hilar – relating to a hilum

Hilum (of the lung) – the point at which the bronchi, pulmonary arteries and veins, lymphatic vessels and nerves enter the lung

Homogenous – uniform in structure or composition throughout

Horner's syndrome – a clinical syndrome consisting of ipsilateral ptosis, miosis and anhidrosis caused by damage to the cervical sympathetic nervous system

Hyperinflation – the lung volume is abnormally increased, with increased filling of the alveoli

Hypertension – high blood pressure

Hypotension – low blood pressure

Hypoxia – a pathological condition in which the body or a tissue is deprived of adequate oxygen supply

Iatrogenic – due to the action of a doctor or a therapy the doctor prescribed

Idiopathic pulmonary fibrosis – a chronic, progressive form of lung disease characterised by fibrosis of the lungs and where the cause is unknown

Immunosuppressed – lacking a fully effective immune system

Infarct – an area of tissue death (necrosis) due to a lack of oxygen, caused by an obstruction of the tissue's blood supply

Inferior – lower in place or position, the opposite of superior

Inspiration – breathing in

Interlobular – between lobules

Interstitial – relating to the interstitium

Interstitium – the space between cells in a tissue

Ionisation – the process in which a neutral atom or molecule gains or loses electrons and thus acquires a negative or positive electrical charge. Ionising radiation produces ionisation in its passage through body tissue or other matter. Ionisation can also cause cell death or mutation (*pleural:* ***ionisations***)

IRMER 2000 – The Ionising Radiation (Medical Exposure) Regulations 2000. Introduced in 2000, it lays down the basic measures for radiation protection for patients

Laparoscopy – a type of minimally invasive surgery in which a small incision (cut) is made in the abdominal wall through which an instrument called a laparoscope is inserted to permit structures within the abdomen and pelvis to be seen

Laparotomy – a surgical procedure involving a large incision through the abdominal wall to gain access to the abdominal cavity

Lateral – situated at the side; away from the middle; extending away from the median plane of the body

Left atrial appendage – part of the left atrium as seen on a PA chest X-ray

Lesion – a general term referring to almost any abnormality involving any tissue or organ

Lingula – a projection of the left upper lobe that closely opposes the left heart border

Lobar – relating to a lobe

Lobe – a clear anatomical division of the lung that can be determined without the use of a microscope, e.g. the left lung is comprised of two lobes and the right lung is comprised of three lobes

Lobectomy – an operation to remove a lobe of the lung

Lobular – relating to a lobule

Lobulated – made up of lobules

Lobule – in contrast to a lobe, lobules are clear anatomical divisions only visible under a microscope

Lumen – the inner open space or cavity of a tube, e.g. blood vessel, intestine or a cannula

Lymph – an almost colourless fluid that travels through lymphatic vessels in the lymphatic system and carries cells that help fight infection and disease

Lymph glands – small glands found throughout the body; they are a part of the lymphatic system and play a major role in the immune system

Lymphadenopathy – abnormally enlarged lymph nodes

Lymphangitis carcinomatosa – inflammation of the lymphatics secondary to a malignancy

Lymphatics – small vessels that collect and carry lymph from the body to ultimately drain back into the bloodstream

Lysis – breakdown of a cell

Magnetic resonance imaging (MRI) – a medical imaging technique that does not use ionising radiation, but magnetic fields and radio frequency fields to produce an image of a detailed cross-section of tissue

Mainstem bronchus – one of the two main branches of the trachea. The trachea splits at the carina to give the right mainstem bronchus and left mainstem bronchus

Malignancy – cancerous cells that have the ability to spread to other sites in the body (metastasise) or to invade and destroy tissues

Medial – situated in the middle; extending towards the middle; closer to the middle/median plane of the body

Median sternotomy wires – metal sutures used to close the sternum after a median sternotomy is performed during open heart surgery

Mediastinal – relating to the mediastinum

Mediastinum – the central compartment of the thoracic cavity. It contains the heart, the great vessels, oesophagus, trachea, phrenic nerve, vagus nerve, sympathetic chain, thoracic duct, thymus and central lymph nodes (including hilar lymph nodes)

Meniscus – the concave upper surface of a liquid

Metastasis – the process by which a cancer spreads from the place at which it first arose as a primary tumour to distant locations in the body; the cancer resulting from the spread of the primary tumour

Metastatic – relating to metastasis

Microbiology – the laboratory department studying microorganisms, e.g. the presence and type of bacteria in a pleural fluid aspirate

Mitotic – relating to cell division

MRI – *see* **Magnetic resonance imaging**

Mucus – secretions produced in the bronchial tubes to remove foreign particles from the lung

Mutation – a change in the structure of the genes or chromosomes of an organism

Nasogastric (NG) – referring to the passage from the nose to the stomach

Nasogastric (NG) tube – a tube that is passed through the nose down into the stomach

Neoplasm – an abnormal mass of tissue due to the abnormal proliferation of cells. They may be benign or malignant

Neurofibroma – a tumour, usually benign, that consists of nerve fibres and connective tissue, caused by an abnormal proliferation of Schwann cells (*pleural: neurofibromata*)

NG – *see* **Nasogastric**

Nodular shadowing – small discrete opacities 1–5 mm in diameter, may be seen on a chest radiograph in patients with fibrosis

Nuclear medicine – the branch or specialty of medicine and medical imaging that uses radionuclides and relies on the process of radioactive decay in the diagnosis and treatment of disease

Oblique – situated in a slanting position

Oedema – *see* **Dependent oedema**

Oligaemia (pulmonary) – deficiency in the volume of blood; reduced circulating intravascular volume

Opacity – an opaque or non-transparent area (*pleural: opacities*)

Organogenesis – the formation and development or organs

PA (posterior–anterior) – the X-ray tube is placed behind the patient and the X-rays pass in the posterior–anterior direction

Pacemaker – a small electronic device that is placed in the chest to help control abnormal heart rhythms

PACS – *see* **Picture archiving and communication system**

Paediatric – relating to children

Pancoast tumour – a type of lung cancer defined by its location at the apex of the lung

Pancoast's syndrome – pain and muscle atrophy in the upper limb due to a Pancoast tumour invading the brachial plexus

Paratracheal – adjacent to the trachea

Parenchyma – the functional parts of an organ in the body. This is in contrast to the stroma, which refers to the structural tissue of organs, namely the connective tissues

Parietal pleura – *see* **Pleura**

PE – *see* **Pulmonary embolism**

Pectoralis major – a thick, fan-shaped muscle situated on the anterior chest wall

Percussion – an assessment method in which the surface of the body is struck with the fingertips to obtain sounds that can be heard or vibrations that can be felt

Peri-bronchial – adjacent to the bronchus

Peri-hilar – adjacent to the hilum

Periphery – the outermost boundary of an area; the surface of an object (*pleural: peripheries*)

Peritoneal cavity – the interior of the peritoneum, the lining of the abdominal cavity

PET – *see* **Positron emission tomography**

Phrenic nerve – the nervous supply to the diaphragm originating from C3-5

Picture archiving and communication system (PACS) – a computer-based digital film storage system for storing X-ray images, thereby eliminating the need for film

Plaques – *see* **Asbestos plaques**

Pleura – a serous membrane that folds back onto itself to form a two-layered membrane structure. The thin space between the two pleural layers is known as the pleural cavity; it normally contains a small amount of pleural fluid. The outer pleura (**parietal pleura**) is attached to the chest wall. The inner pleura (**visceral pleura**) covers the lungs and adjoining structures

Pleural effusion – a condition that results from fluid accumulating in the pleural cavity

Pleural space (Pleural cavity) – *see* **Pleura**

Pleurisy – inflammation of the pleura occurring when an infection or damaging agent irritates the pleural surface. As a consequence, the patient may develop sharp chest pains

Pleuritic pain – pain relating to pleurisy

Pneumoconiosis – an occupational lung disease caused by the inhalation of dust, often in mines. One of the causes of lung fibrosis

Pneumonectomy – an operation to remove a lung

Pneumonia – an inflammatory condition of the lung, often due to infection

Pneumoperitoneum – air or gas in the abdominal (peritoneal) cavity

Pneumothorax – a collection of air or gas in the pleural cavity of the chest

Positron emission tomography – a nuclear medicine imaging method similar to computed tomography, except that the image shows the tissue concentration of a positron-emitting radioisotope

Posterior – located behind or towards the rear of a structure

Projection – the X-ray view, i.e. AP, PA, supine or lateral

Pulmonary – relating to the lungs

Pulmonary embolism (PE) – a blockage of one of the main arteries of the lung or one of its branches by a substance (embolus) that has travelled from elsewhere in the body through the bloodstream (usually a thrombus)

Pulmonary hypertension – high blood pressure in the pulmonary arteries that convey blood from the right ventricle to the lungs

Pulmonary oedema – a diffuse extravascular accumulation of fluid in the pulmonary tissues and air spaces due to changes in hydrostatic forces in the capillaries or to increased capillary permeability

Pus – a yellowish-white fluid formed in infected tissue, consisting of white blood cells, cellular debris and necrotic tissue

Radiation – the transfer of energy in the form of particles or waves

Radiosensitive – sensitive to the biological effects of radiant energy such as X-rays

Radiotherapy – the treatment of disease using radiation directed at the body from an external source or emitted by radioactive materials placed within the body

Reticular shadowing – a fine or coarse branching linear pattern produced by thickening of the lung interstitium (connective tissue). The heart loses its normal smooth outline and seems 'shaggy'. It may be seen on a chest radiograph in patients with fibrosis

Reticulonodular shadowing – a mixture of reticular-type shadowing and nodular-type shadowing. Seen on a chest radiograph in patients with fibrosis

Retroperitoneal – situated behind the peritoneum

Rotation – the circular movement of an object around a point or centre of rotation

Sarcoidosis – a disease of unknown origin marked by the formation of granulomatous lesions that may appear in many organs, especially in the liver, lungs, skin and lymph nodes. One of the causes of lung fibrosis

Sarcoma – a malignant tumour derived from connective tissue

Septal lines – the radiographic appearance of engorgement of the pulmonary interlobular septal lymphatics. They are seen around the periphery of the lungs, extending inwards from the pleural surface. They are invisible on the normal chest radiograph and only become visible when thickened by fluid, tumour or fibrosis

Septum – a thin partition or membrane that divides two cavities or soft masses of tissue in an organism

Shadowing – *see* **Opacity**

Shock – a medical emergency in which the organs and tissues of the body are not receiving an adequate flow of blood

Silhouette – an outline that appears dark against a light background or light against a dark background

SLE – *see* **Systemic lupus erythematosus**

Spiculated – spiky

Spinous process – the part of each vertebrae projecting backwards giving attachment to the back muscles

Squamous cell carcinoma – a form of bronchial carcinoma, usually in middle-aged smokers

Stenotic – a structure that is narrowed or strictured

Sternotomy wires – *see* **Median sternotomy wires**

Subcutaneous – just beneath the skin

Subcutaneous emphysema – when air or gas is present in the subcutaneous layer of the skin

Subphrenic – the area under the diaphragm

Superior – higher in place or position, the opposite of inferior

Supine – lying on the back with face upwards

Surfactant – a substance produced by alveolar cells of the lung to maintain stability of the pulmonary tissue by lowering the surface tension of fluids that coat the lung

Surgical emphysema – *see* **Subcutaneous emphysema**

Sympathetic chain – a paired bundle of nerve fibres that run from the base of the skull to the coccyx

Systemic lupus erythematosus (SLE) – a systemic autoimmune disease that can affect any part of the body. It is one of the causes of lung fibrosis

Systemic sclerosis – a systemic autoimmune connective tissue disease. One of the causes of lung fibrosis

TB – *see* **Tuberculosis**

Tension pneumothorax – a serious type of pneumothorax whereby air enters, but cannot leave, the pleural space. This can lead to a complete collapse of the lung and is a medical emergency. It should be a clinical diagnosis

Thoracic duct – the largest lymphatic vessel in the body, it starts in the abdomen and runs superiorly, ascending the posterior mediastinum before draining into the systemic circulation via the left brachiocephalic vein

Thoracoplasty – a former treatment for pulmonary tuberculosis involving surgical removal of parts of the ribs, thus allowing the chest wall to fall in and collapse the affected lung

Thoracotomy – surgical opening of the chest cavity to inspect or operate on the heart, lungs or other structures within

Thorax – the chest

Thymic – relating to the thymus

Thymus – a lymphoid organ situated in the centre of the upper chest just behind the sternum (breastbone)

Thyroid – a large endocrine gland situated in the neck

Tissue – an aggregation of similarly specialised cells which together perform certain special functions

Trachea – windpipe

Transudate – an extravascular fluid with low protein content (<30 g/l of protein)

Tuberculoma – a tumour-like mass resulting from a localised tuberculosis infection

Tuberculosis – a potentially fatal contagious disease that can affect almost any part of the body but is mainly an infection of the lungs. It is caused by the mycobacterium *Mycobacterium tuberculosis*

Tumour – an abnormal swelling or mass of tissue

Ultrasound – a diagnostic medical imaging technique using ultrasound waves to visualise subcutaneous body structures

Usual interstitial pneumonitis – a form of lung disease characterised by progressive fibrosis of both lungs

Vagus nerve – the 10th cranial nerve, passing through the neck and thorax into the abdomen and supplying sensation to part of the ear, the tongue, the larynx and the pharynx, motor impulses to the vocal cords, and motor and secretory impulses to the abdominal and thoracic viscera

Visceral pleura – *see* **Pleura**

Index

Page numbers in *italic* denote figures.

Chest X-rays for Medical Students, First Edition. Christopher Clarke, Anthony Dux.
© 2011 John Wiley & Sons, Ltd. Published 2011 by Blackwell Publishing Ltd.